I0772456

THE ULTIMATE SMOOTHIE CLEANSE FOR BEGINNERS

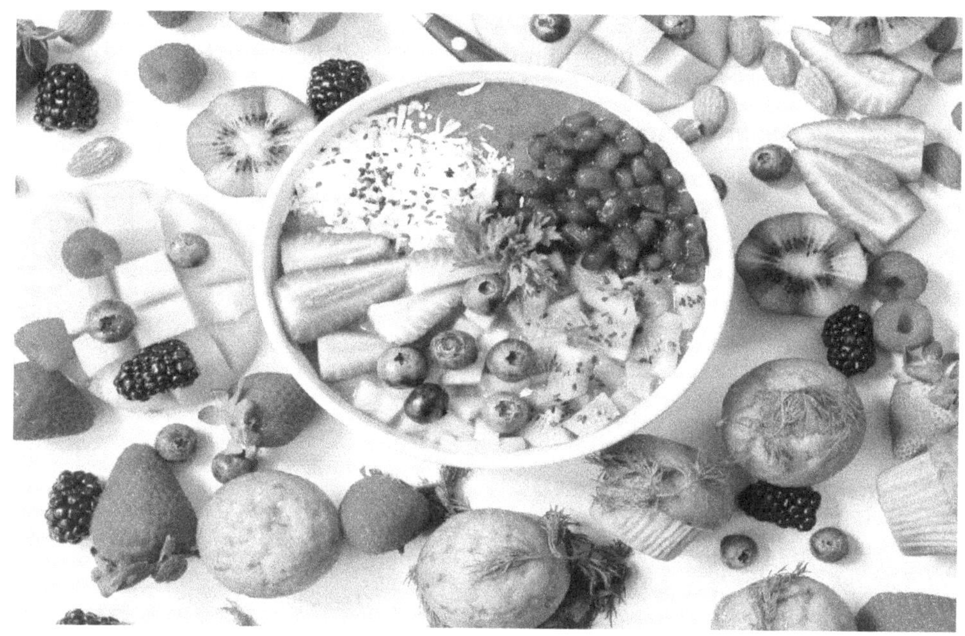

A Guide to Detoxing and Rejuvenating Your Body

Lani Williams

Copyright © 2023 Lani Williams

All rights reserved. No part of this book may be reproduced, stored, or transmitted by any means—whether auditory, graphic, mechanical, or electronic—without written permission of both the copyright owner and the above publisher of this book. Unauthorized reproduction of any part of this work is illegal and is punishable by law.

This book is a work of non-fiction and is intended to be factual. All names, characters, places, and incidents are the product of the author's imagination or are used fictitiously. Any resemblance to actual persons, living or dead, events, or locales is entirely coincidental.

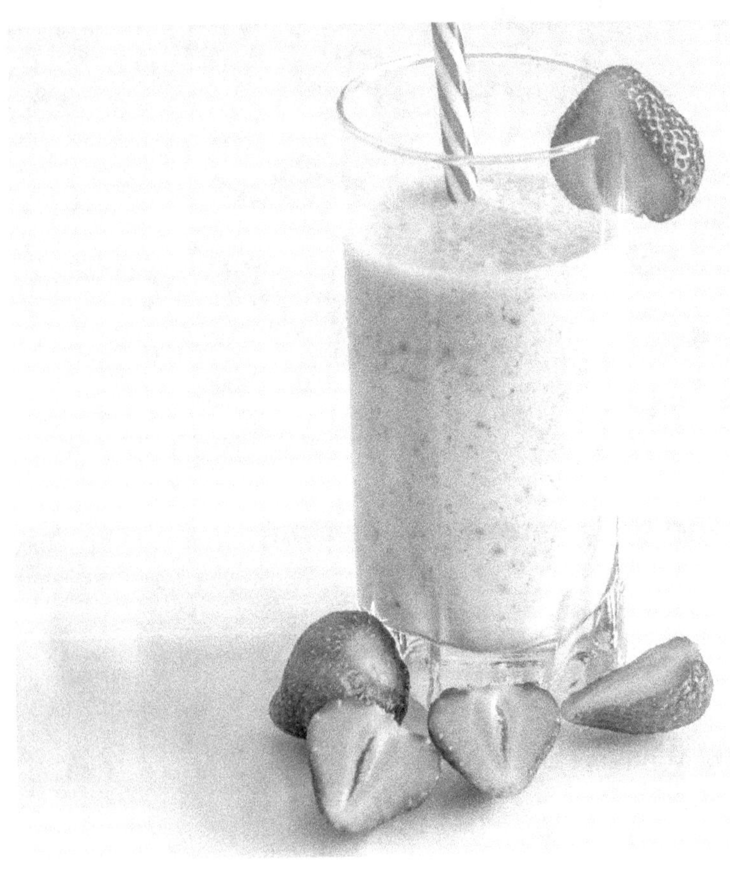

TABLE OF CONTENTS

INTRODUCTION

Once upon a time, there was a health-conscious woman who felt like she was stuck in a rut. She was feeling sluggish and was desperate to find a way to become energized again. After doing some research, she stumbled upon the idea of a smoothie cleanse.

The smoothie cleanse seemed like a great way to jumpstart her diet and detoxify her body, but she had no idea where to start. That's when she discovered a book online for beginners like her.

This book offered her an easy-to-follow guide for transitioning to a healthier lifestyle through the power of smoothies.

The woman was so excited to start her journey to a healthier life that she read the book from cover to cover. She was amazed at how much she learned about the benefits of smoothies, and how simple the recipes were to follow.

She had finally found the perfect way to jumpstart her health journey and felt more energized than ever before. And now, she wants to share her story and recipes with you! Inside the Ultimate Smoothie Cleanse for Beginners, you'll find over 50 delicious smoothie recipes, along with helpful tips and tricks to make your cleanse a success.

So, if you're ready to take your health and wellness to the next level, let the Ultimate Smoothie Cleanse for Beginners help you get there!

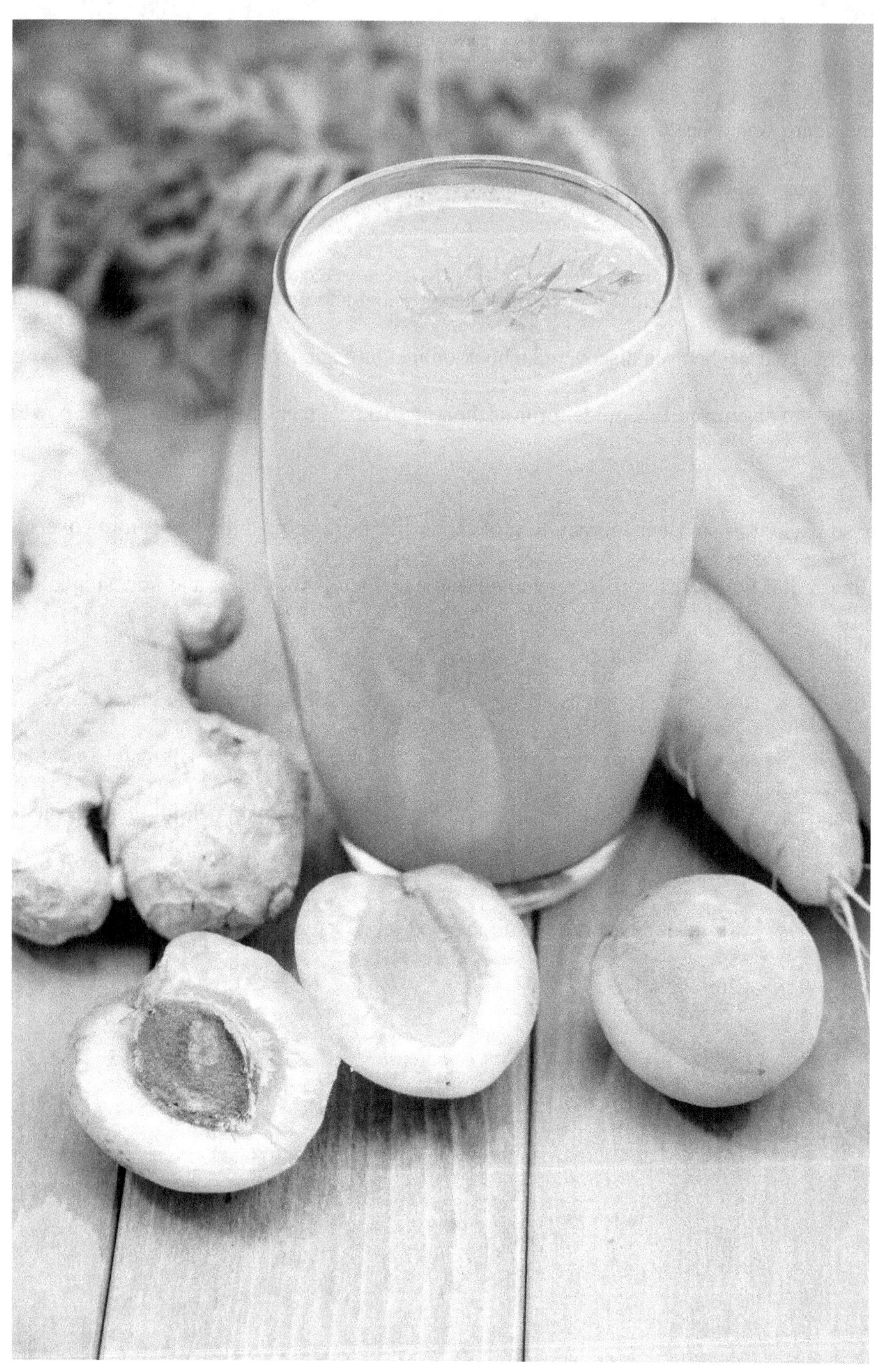

INTRODUCTION TO SMOOTHIE CLEANSE

A smoothie cleanse is an effective way to detoxify and reset your body. It involves replacing meals with smoothies made from fresh fruits and vegetables. This type of detoxification can help to flush out toxins, reduce inflammation, and improve digestion.

Smoothies are a great way to get a nutrient-dense meal in a short amount of time. They are simple to prepare and can be consumed at any time of day. They are also a great way to get your daily dose of fruits and veggies without having to spend too much time preparing meals.

A smoothie cleanse involves replacing one or more meals a day with a smoothie. The basic idea is to consume a nutrient-dense smoothie that is low in sugar and calories, but high in vitamins, minerals, antioxidants, and fiber. This type of cleanse can be done for a few days to a few weeks, depending on your individual needs.

When designing your smoothie cleanse, it is important to include a variety of fruits and vegetables. You can use fresh fruits and vegetables, or frozen ones if you prefer. Some of the most popular ingredients for smoothies include bananas, berries, spinach, kale, and avocado. You can also add nuts, seeds, nut butters, and plant-based milks for extra nutrients and flavor.

It is also important to make sure that you are drinking plenty of water. Aim for at least eight 8-ounce glasses of water each day. This will help ensure that your body is properly hydrated and that you are getting all the nutrients and benefits from your smoothie.

Before beginning a smoothie cleanse, it is important to consult with your doctor. This is especially important for those with certain medical conditions or who are pregnant or nursing. Your doctor can provide guidance on the best approach to take.

With a little bit of planning, you can create a nutrient-dense smoothie that will give your body the reset it needs.

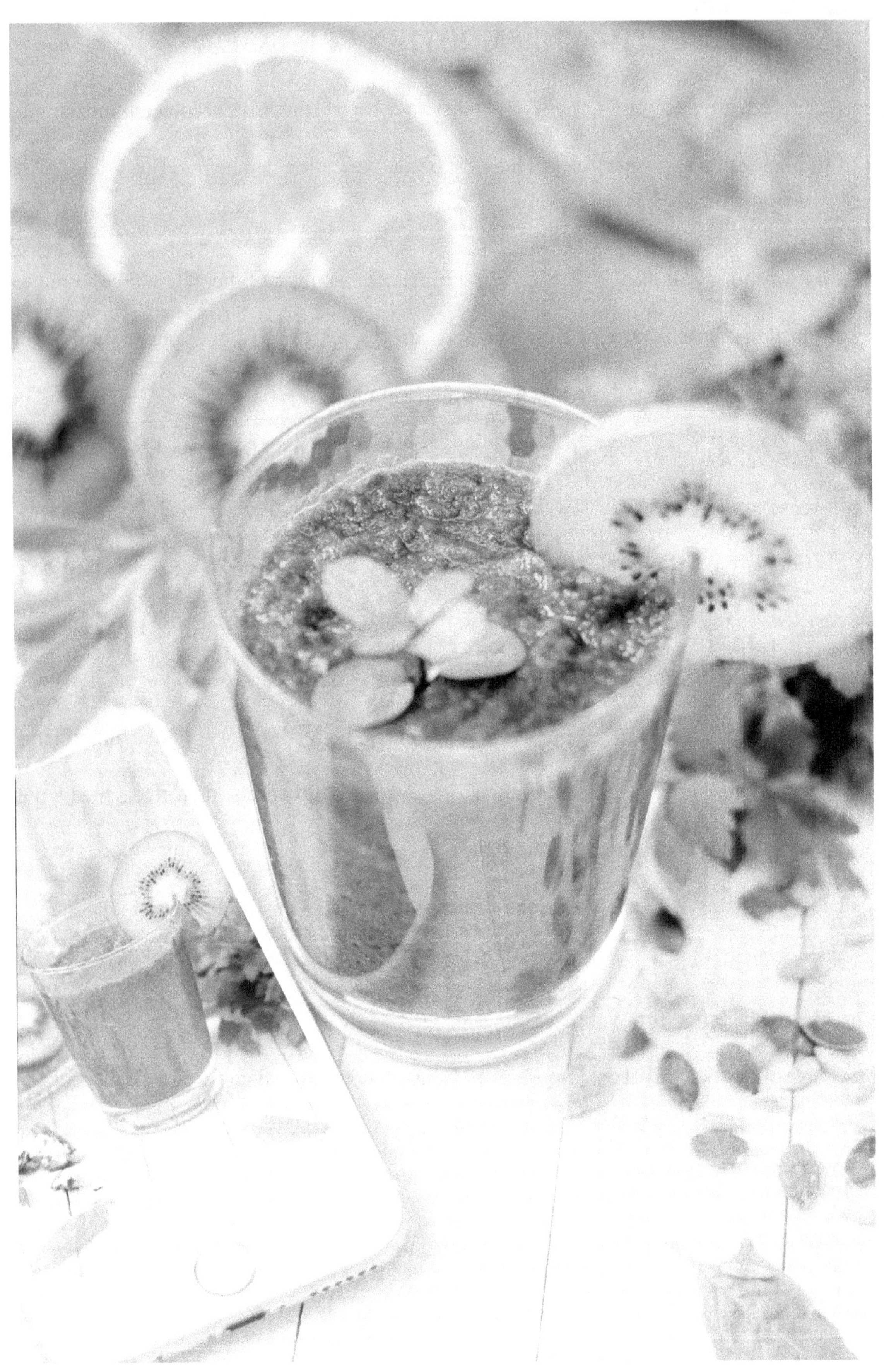

PART 1: PREPPING FOR A SMOOTHIE CLEANSE

BENEFITS OF SMOOTHIE CLEANSING

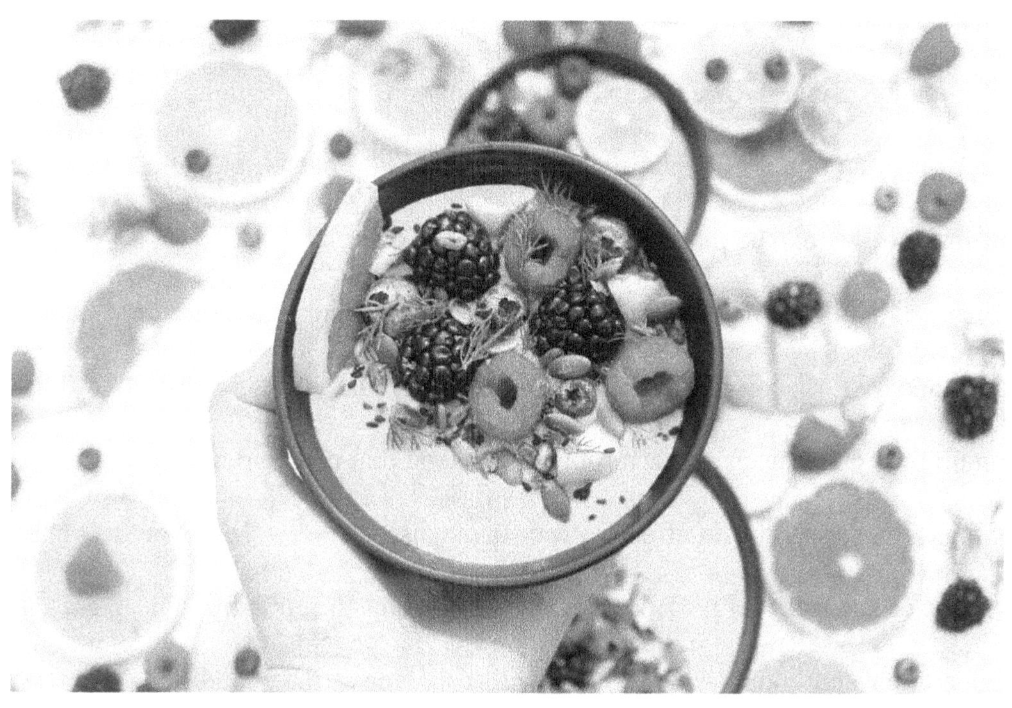

A smoothie cleanse is a type of diet that involves consuming only smoothies for a specific period of time. This type of diet has become increasingly popular in recent years as people look for ways to improve their health and lose weight. There are many potential benefits of following a smoothie cleanse.

1. Detoxification: Smoothie cleanses can help your body detoxify and rid itself of toxins. Many of the ingredients used in smoothies, such as fruits and vegetables, contain antioxidants, vitamins, and minerals that help to flush out toxins from the body. Additionally, some smoothie cleanses include the use of herbs and spices that can aid in detoxification.

2. Weight Loss: Smoothie cleanses can help you lose weight. Since the drinks are low in calories and high in nutrients, they can help you feel fuller for longer periods of time. Additionally, many smoothies contain metabolism-boosting ingredients such as matcha green tea and ginger that can help you burn fat.

3. Improved Digestion: Smoothies are high in fiber and water, which can help improve your digestion. Fiber helps to move food through the digestive tract, and water encourages the body to flush out toxins. Additionally, some smoothies contain probiotics, which are beneficial bacteria that help to break down food and aid in digestion.

4. Improved Immunity: Smoothies are packed with vitamins and minerals that can help boost your immune system. Many smoothies contain ingredients such as spinach, kale, and blueberries, which are all high in antioxidants that can help protect your body from disease.

5. Increased Energy: Smoothies are a great source of energy. Many of the ingredients used in smoothies, such as bananas and yogurt, contain natural sugars that provide an energy boost. Additionally, some smoothies contain ingredients such as maca root and ginseng that can help increase energy levels.

Overall, smoothie cleanses can be an effective way to cleanse the body, lose weight, improve digestion, boost immunity, and increase energy. However, it is important to remember that these cleanses should be used in moderation and should be followed with a balanced diet. Additionally, it is important to consult your doctor before beginning a smoothie cleanse to make sure that it is safe for you.

UNDERSTANDING SMOOTHIE CLEANSE INGREDIENTS

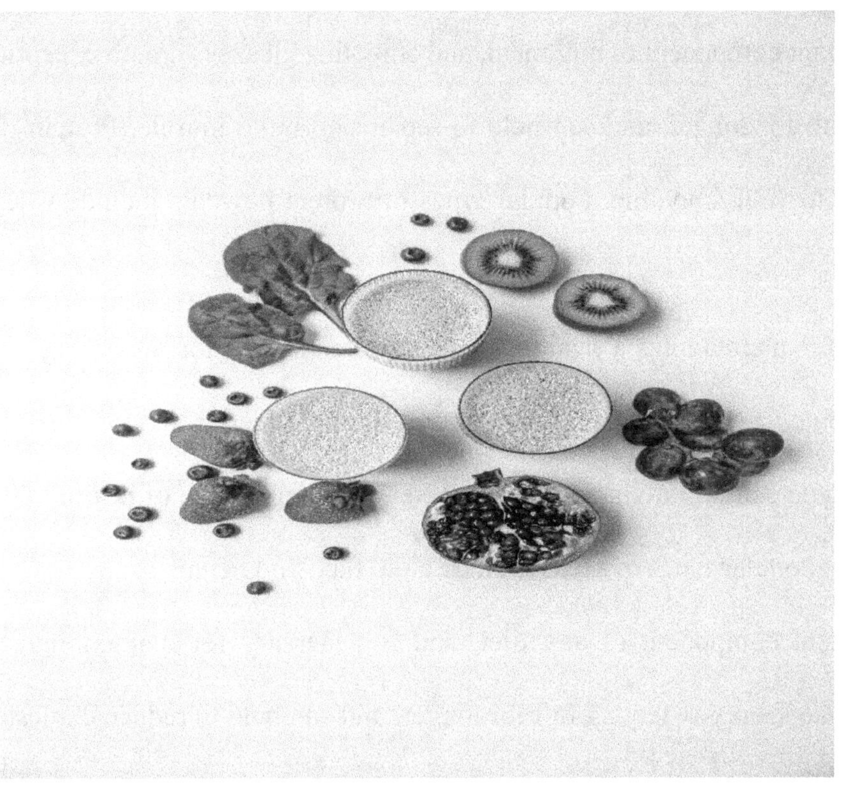

It can be difficult to understand all the different ingredients that go into a smoothie cleanse and how they work together to create a nutritious meal as a beginner.

So, let's examine some of the most common ingredients found in smoothie cleanses and how they work together to provide health benefits.

The most important ingredient in a smoothie cleanse is the base. This is usually a liquid like water, almond milk, coconut milk, or juice. The base provides the bulk of the liquid in the smoothie, and helps to create a smooth texture. It also helps to thin out the other ingredients, allowing them to blend together easily.

Fruits and vegetables are essential for any smoothie cleanse. Fruits provide natural sweetness, vitamins, minerals, and fiber. Popular fruits used in smoothie cleanses include bananas, strawberries, blueberries, apples, oranges, and pineapples. Vegetables provide a different type of nutrition, including vitamins, minerals, and antioxidants. Common vegetables used in smoothie cleanses are kale, spinach, carrots, beets, and cucumber.

Protein is an important component of any meal, and smoothie cleanses are no exception. Protein helps to keep you feeling full for longer, and can help to repair and build muscle. Protein powders are a great way to add protein to your smoothie. Popular types of protein powders include whey, plant-based, and hemp.

Fats are essential for maintaining a healthy diet, and are needed for absorbing certain vitamins and minerals. Healthy fats, such as nuts and nut butters, can be added to a smoothie cleanse to provide a source of energy and essential fatty acids. Seeds are also a great source of healthy fats and can be easily added to smoothies. Popular types of seeds include chia, flax, and hemp.

Fiber is an important component of any diet, and is necessary for maintaining a healthy digestive system. Fiber helps to keep you feeling full for longer, and can help to reduce cholesterol levels. Popular sources of fiber for smoothies are oats, chia seeds, and flax seeds.

Finally, sweeteners can be added to smoothies to give them a sweeter taste. Natural sweeteners, such as honey and maple syrup, are a great way to add sweetness without using refined sugar.

By understanding the different components of a smoothie cleanse and how they work together, you can create a nutritious and delicious smoothie that will help you reach your health goals. By adding a variety of fruits, vegetables, proteins, fats, fibers, and sweeteners, you can create a balanced and nutritious meal that will provide you with the essential vitamins and minerals needed for a healthy lifestyle.

SHOPPING LIST AND KITCHEN SET-UP

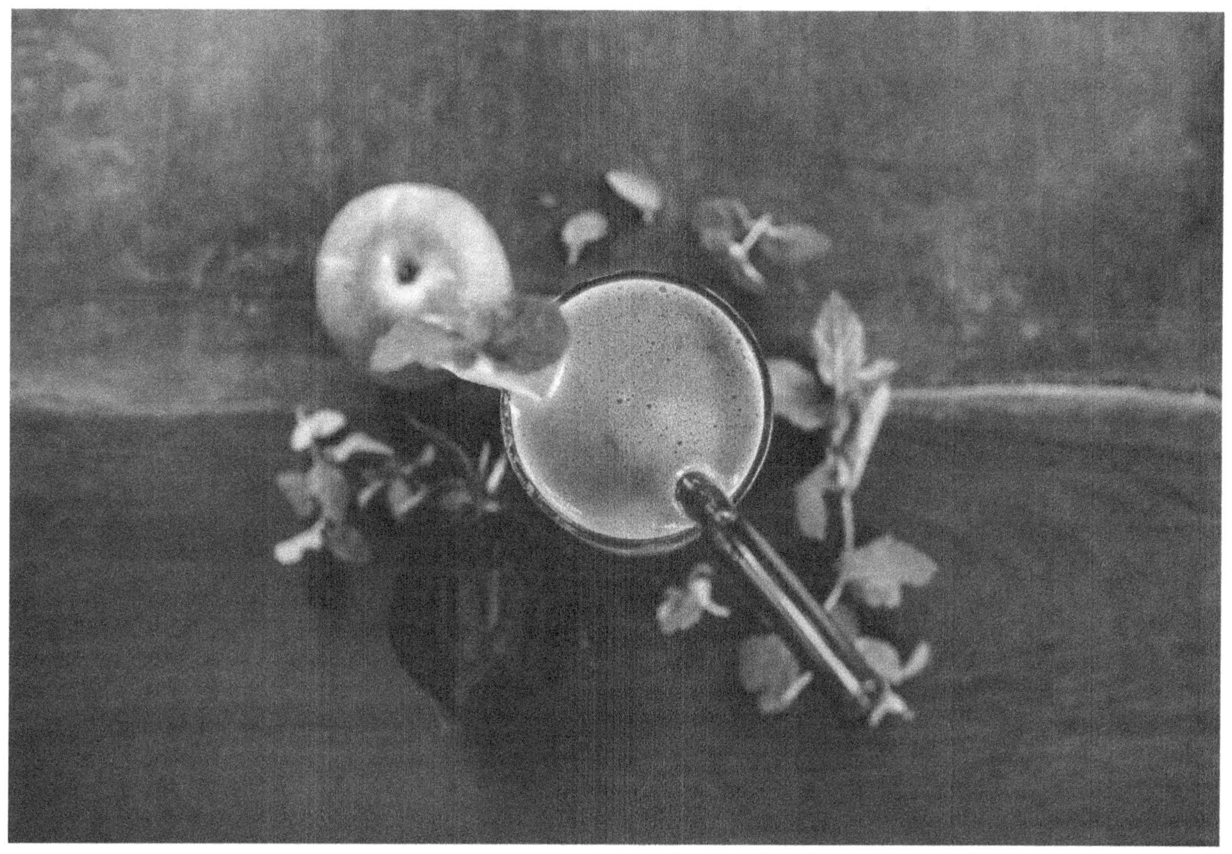

The first step in any smoothie cleanse is stocking up on the right ingredients. This doesn't have to be an intimidating task; if you're just starting out, it's best to focus on the basics. Here's a list of ingredients you'll need for a beginner's smoothie cleanse:

-Fruits: Bananas, apples, oranges, strawberries, blueberries, mangoes, and more

-Vegetables: Spinach, kale, cucumber, carrots, celery, and more

-Protein: Greek yogurt, milk, nut butters, chia seeds, hemp seeds, and more

-Fats: Coconut milk, avocado, nut butters, and more

-Sweeteners: Honey, maple syrup, dates, and more

-Superfoods: Spirulina, chlorella, goji berries, maca powder, and more

Kitchen Set-up

Once your grocery list is complete, it's time to make sure your kitchen is set up for success. Here are some kitchen essentials you'll need for a successful smoothie cleanse:

-Blender: A good blender is essential for blending your ingredients into a tasty, smooth smoothie.

-Storage containers: You'll need to store your ingredients in the fridge and freezer, so having a few good storage containers on hand will make the process easier.

-Sharp knives: You'll need sharp knives to cut up your fruits and vegetables.

-Cutting board: Having a cutting board will make prepping your ingredients much easier.

-Measuring cups and spoons: You'll need these to measure out the right amount of your ingredients.

 With a little grocery shopping, kitchen set-up, and smoothie recipes, you'll be ready to start your smoothie cleanse in no time.

Once you've got your kitchen set up and your ingredients ready, it's time to start making your smoothies!

PART 2: SMOOTHIE CLEANSE RECIPES

BREAKFAST SMOOTHIES

Breakfast smoothies are a great way to start the day. They provide a healthy and nutritious meal in a convenient package. Smoothies are filled with fiber, vitamins, and minerals, and can be tailored to provide tailored nutrition. Plus, they are easy to make, and can be taken on the go. Start your day right with a nutritious breakfast smoothie, and you'll be set for a productive day.

1. Banana Oatmeal Breakfast Smoothie:

Ingredients: 1 ripe banana, 1/2 cup oats, 1 cup almond milk, 1/2 teaspoon cinnamon, 1/2 teaspoon ground nutmeg

Instructions: In a blender, combine all of the ingredients and blend until desired consistency. Pour into a glass and enjoy! Prep time: 5 minutes

2. Strawberry Banana Breakfast Smoothie:

Ingredients: 1 ripe banana, 1 cup strawberries, 1/2 cup plain Greek yogurt, 1/4 cup honey, 1 cup almond milk

Instructions: In a blender, combine all of the ingredients and blend until desired consistency. Pour into a glass and enjoy! Prep time: 5 minutes

3. Blueberry Peach Breakfast Smoothie:

Ingredients: 1/2 cup blueberries, 1/2 cup sliced peaches, 1/2 cup Greek yogurt, 1/4 cup honey, 1 cup almond milk

Instructions: In a blender, combine all of the ingredients and blend until desired consistency. Pour into a glass and enjoy! Prep time: 5 minutes

4. Mango Coconut Breakfast Smoothie:

Ingredients: 1/2 cup mango, 1/4 cup coconut flakes, 1/2 cup Greek yogurt, 1/4 cup honey, 1 cup almond milk

Instructions: In a blender, combine all of the ingredients and blend until desired consistency. Pour into a glass and enjoy! Prep time: 5 minutes

5. Avocado Spinach Breakfast Smoothie:

Ingredients: 1/2 ripe avocado, 1/2 cup spinach, 1/2 cup plain Greek yogurt, 1/4 cup honey, 1 cup almond milk

Instructions: In a blender, combine all of the ingredients and blend until desired consistency. Pour into a glass and enjoy! Prep time: 5 minutes

6. Pineapple Coconut Breakfast Smoothie:

Ingredients: 1/2 cup pineapple, 1/4 cup coconut flakes, 1/2 cup plain Greek yogurt, 1/4 cup honey, 1 cup almond milk

Instructions: In a blender, combine all of the ingredients and blend until desired consistency. Pour into a glass and enjoy! Prep time: 5 minutes

7. Pomegranate Chia Breakfast Smoothie:

Ingredients: 1/2 cup pomegranate seeds, 1 tablespoon chia seeds, 1/2 cup plain Greek yogurt, 1/4 cup honey, 1 cup almond milk

Instructions: In a blender, combine all of the ingredients and blend until desired consistency. Pour into a glass and enjoy! Prep time: 5 minutes

8. Peach Coconut Breakfast Smoothie:

Ingredients: 1/2 cup sliced peaches, 1/4 cup coconut flakes, 1/2 cup plain Greek yogurt, 1/4 cup honey, 1 cup almond milk

Instructions: In a blender, combine all of the ingredients and blend until desired consistency. Pour into a glass and enjoy! Prep time: 5 minutes

9. Apple Cinnamon Breakfast Smoothie:

Ingredients: 1/2 cup diced apples, 1/2 teaspoon cinnamon, 1/2 cup plain Greek yogurt, 1/4 cup honey, 1 cup almond milk

Instructions: In a blender, combine all of the ingredients and blend until desired consistency. Pour into a glass and enjoy! Prep time: 5 minutes

10. Raspberry Coconut Breakfast Smoothie:

Ingredients: 1/2 cup raspberries, 1/4 cup coconut flakes, 1/2 cup plain Greek yogurt, 1/4 cup honey, 1 cup almond milk

Instructions: In a blender, combine all of the ingredients and blend until desired consistency. Pour into a glass and enjoy! Prep time: 5 minutes

11. Banana Walnut Breakfast Smoothie:

Ingredients: 1 ripe banana, 2 tablespoons walnuts, 1/2 cup plain Greek yogurt, 1/4 cup honey, 1 cup almond milk

Instructions: In a blender, combine all of the ingredients and blend until desired consistency. Pour into a glass and enjoy! Prep time: 5 minutes

12. Date Coconut Breakfast Smoothie:

Ingredients: 1/4 cup pitted dates, 1/4 cup coconut flakes, 1/2 cup plain Greek yogurt, 1/4 cup honey, 1 cup almond milk

Instructions: In a blender, combine all of the ingredients and blend until desired consistency. Pour into a glass and enjoy! Prep time: 5 minutes

13. Kale Banana Breakfast Smoothie:

Ingredients: 1/2 cup kale, 1 ripe banana, 1/2 cup plain Greek yogurt, 1/4 cup honey, 1 cup almond milk

Instructions: In a blender, combine all of the ingredients and blend until desired consistency. Pour into a glass and enjoy! Prep time: 5 minutes

14. Mango Chia Breakfast Smoothie:

Ingredients: 1/2 cup mango, 1 tablespoon chia seeds, 1/2 cup plain Greek yogurt, 1/4 cup honey, 1 cup almond milk

Instructions: In a blender, combine all of the ingredients and blend until desired consistency. Pour into a glass and enjoy! Prep time: 5 minutes

15. Strawberry Flaxseed Breakfast Smoothie:

Ingredients: 1 cup strawberries, 1 tablespoon flaxseeds, 1/2 cup plain Greek yogurt, 1/4 cup honey, 1 cup almond milk

Instructions: In a blender, combine all of the ingredients and blend until desired consistency. Pour into a glass and enjoy! Prep time: 5 minutes

PROTEIN SMOOTHIES

Protein smoothies are a great way to get protein in a convenient and delicious form. The protein helps to build and repair muscle, which can help improve physical performance. They also provide sustained energy, making them a great snack or post-workout drink. Protein smoothies are also a great way to get essential vitamins, minerals and other nutrients. They're easy to make and can be customized to fit any dietary needs. Enjoy them anytime for a quick and nutritious boost!

1. Blueberry-Banana Protein Smoothie

– Prep Time: 5 minutes

Ingredients:

• ½ cup almond milk

• ½ cup plain Greek yogurt

• ½ banana

• ½ cup blueberries

• 1 scoop of vanilla protein powder

• 1 teaspoon honey

Instructions:

1. Combine all ingredients in a blender and blend until desired consistency.

2. Pour and enjoy!

2. Peanut Butter & Chocolate Protein Smoothie

– Prep Time: 5 minutes

Ingredients:

• ¾ cup almond milk

• 2 tablespoons peanut butter

• 1 tablespoon cocoa powder

• 1 banana

• 1 scoop of chocolate protein powder

• 2-3 ice cubes

Instructions:

1. Combine all ingredients in a blender and blend until desired consistency.

2. Pour and enjoy!

3. Strawberry-Kiwi Protein Smoothie

– Prep Time: 5 minutes

Ingredients:

• ½ cup almond milk

• ½ cup plain Greek yogurt

• ½ cup strawberries

• 1 kiwi

• 1 scoop of vanilla protein powder

• 2-3 ice cubes

Instructions:

1. Combine all ingredients in a blender and blend until desired consistency.

2. Pour and enjoy!

4. Coconut-Mango Protein Smoothie

– Prep Time: 5 minutes

Ingredients:

- ½ cup coconut milk

- ½ cup plain Greek yogurt

- ½ cup mango

- 1 scoop of vanilla protein powder

- 2 tablespoons honey

Instructions:

1. Combine all ingredients in a blender and blend until desired consistency.

2. Pour and enjoy!

5. Avocado-Pineapple Protein Smoothie

– Prep Time: 5 minutes

Ingredients:

- ½ cup almond milk

- ½ cup plain Greek yogurt

- ½ avocado

- ½ cup pineapple

- 1 scoop of vanilla protein powder

- 2-3 ice cubes

Instructions:

1. Combine all ingredients in a blender and blend until desired consistency.

2. Pour and enjoy!

6. Orange-Carrot Protein Smoothie

– Prep Time: 5 minutes

Ingredients:

• ½ cup almond milk

• ½ cup plain Greek yogurt

• ½ orange

• ½ cup carrots

• 1 scoop of vanilla protein powder

• 2-3 ice cubes

Instructions:

1. Combine all ingredients in a blender and blend until desired consistency.

2. Pour and enjoy!

7. Apple-Cinnamon Protein Smoothie

– Prep Time: 5 minutes

Ingredients:

• ½ cup almond milk

• ½ cup plain Greek yogurt

• ½ apple

• ½ teaspoon cinnamon

• 1 scoop of vanilla protein powder

• 2-3 ice cubes

Instructions:

1. Combine all ingredients in a blender and blend until desired consistency.

2. Pour and enjoy!

8. Raspberry-Vanilla Protein Smoothie

– Prep Time: 5 minutes

Ingredients:

• ½ cup almond milk

• ½ cup plain Greek yogurt

• ½ cup raspberries

• 1 teaspoon vanilla extract

• 1 scoop of vanilla protein powder

• 2-3 ice cubes

Instructions:

1. Combine all ingredients in a blender and blend until desired consistency.

2. Pour and enjoy!

9. Banana-Cocoa Protein Smoothie

– Prep Time: 5 minutes

Ingredients:

• ½ cup almond milk

• ½ cup plain Greek yogurt

• ½ banana

• 1 tablespoon cocoa powder

• 1 scoop of chocolate protein powder

• 2-3 ice cubes

Instructions:

1. Combine all ingredients in a blender and blend until desired consistency.

2. Pour and enjoy!

10. Almond-Cherry Protein Smoothie

– Prep Time: 5 minutes

Ingredients:

• ½ cup almond milk

• ½ cup plain Greek yogurt

• ¼ cup cherries

• 2 tablespoons almonds

• 1 scoop of vanilla protein powder

• 2-3 ice cubes

Instructions:

1. Combine all ingredients in a blender and blend until desired consistency.

2. Pour and enjoy!

11. Coconut-Banana Protein Smoothie

 – Prep Time: 5 minutes

Ingredients:

• ½ cup coconut milk

• ½ cup plain Greek yogurt

• ½ banana

• 1 scoop of vanilla protein powder

• 2 tablespoons honey

Instructions:

1. Combine all ingredients in a blender and blend until desired consistency.

2. Pour and enjoy!

12. Spinach-Kale Protein Smoothie

– Prep Time: 5 minutes

Ingredients:

• ½ cup almond milk

• ½ cup plain Greek yogurt

• ½ cup spinach

• ½ cup kale

• 1 scoop of vanilla protein powder

• 2-3 ice cubes

Instructions:

1. Combine all ingredients in a blender and blend until desired consistency.

2. Pour and enjoy!

13. Peanut Butter Protein Smoothie

– Prep Time: 5 minutes

Ingredients:

- 1 banana

- 1/2 cup of almond milk

- 2 tablespoons of peanut butter

- 1 scoop of protein powder

- 1 teaspoon of honey

Instructions:

1. Combine all ingredients in a blender and blend until desired consistency.

2. Pour the smoothie into a glass and enjoy!

14. Pineapple-Mango Protein Smoothie

– Prep Time: 5 minutes

Ingredients:

• ½ cup almond milk

• ½ cup plain Greek yogurt

• ½ cup pineapple

• ½ cup mango

• 1 scoop of vanilla protein powder

• 2-3 ice cubes

Instructions:

1. Combine all ingredients in a blender and blend until desired consistency.

2. Pour and enjoy!

15. Peach-Almond Protein Smoothie

– Prep Time :5 minutes

Ingredients:

• ½ cup almond milk

• ½ cup plain Greek yogurt

• ½ cup peaches

• 2 tablespoons almonds

• 1 scoop of vanilla protein powder

• 2-3 ice cubes

Instructions:

1. Combine all ingredients in a blender and blend until desired consistency.

2. Pour and enjoy!

FRUIT SMOOTHIES

Smoothies made from fruits are a healthy and tasty way to start your day. They can provide a boost of energy, essential vitamins and minerals, and are a great way to get your daily intake of fruits. Smoothies are easy to make, can be tailored to individual tastes, are a convenient snack, and can be a satisfying meal replacement. They can help you stay hydrated, aid digestion, and provide a boost of antioxidants.

1. Banana Berry Smoothie

(Prep Time: 5 minutes)

Ingredients:

-2 ripe bananas

-1/2 cup of frozen raspberries

-1/2 cup almond milk

Instructions:

-Add the bananas, frozen raspberries, and almond milk to a blender.

-Blend on high until smooth and creamy.

-Pour into a glass and enjoy!

2. Mango Pineapple Smoothie

 (Prep Time: 5 minutes)

Ingredients:

-1/2 cup fresh or frozen mango

-1/2 cup fresh or frozen pineapple

-1 cup almond milk

Instructions:

-Combine the mango, pineapple, and almond milk in a blender.

-Blend until smooth and creamy.

-Pour into a glass and enjoy!

3. Apple Avocado Smoothie

(Prep Time: 5 minutes)

Ingredients:

-1 apple, cored and chopped

-1/2 avocado, peeled and pitted

-1/2 cup almond milk

Instructions:

-Place the apple, avocado, and almond milk in a blender.

-Blend on high until smooth and creamy.

-Pour into a glass and enjoy!

4. Peach Coconut Smoothie

 (Prep Time: 5 minutes)

Ingredients:

-1 peach, pitted and chopped

-1/4 cup shredded coconut

-1/2 cup almond milk

Instructions:

-Combine the peach, shredded coconut, and almond milk in a blender.

-Blend until smooth and creamy.

-Pour into a glass and enjoy!

5. Orange Kale Smoothie

(Prep Time: 5 minutes)

Ingredients:

-1 orange, peeled and chopped

-1 cup kale, chopped

-1/2 cup almond milk

Instructions:

-Add the orange, kale, and almond milk to a blender.

-Blend on high until smooth and creamy.

-Pour into a glass and enjoy!

6. Pear Ginger Smoothie

(Prep Time: 5 minutes)

Ingredients:

-1 pear, cored and chopped

-1/2 teaspoon ground ginger

-1/2 cup almond milk

Instructions:

-Combine the pear, ground ginger, and almond milk in a blender.

-Blend until smooth and creamy.

-Pour into a glass and enjoy!

7. Kiwi Coconut Smoothie

 (Prep Time: 5 minutes)

Ingredients:

-2 kiwis, peeled and chopped

-1/4 cup shredded coconut

-1/2 cup almond milk

Instructions:

-Add the kiwis, shredded coconut, and almond milk to a blender.

-Blend on high until smooth and creamy.

-Pour into a glass and enjoy!

8. Pineapple Coconut Smoothie

(Prep Time: 5 minutes)

Ingredients:

-1/2 cup fresh or frozen pineapple

-1/4 cup shredded coconut

-1/2 cup almond milk

Instructions:

-Combine the pineapple, shredded coconut, and almond milk in a blender.

-Blend until smooth and creamy.

-Pour into a glass and enjoy!

9. Strawberry Lime Smoothie

(Prep Time: 5 minutes)

Ingredients:

-1/2 cup frozen strawberries

-1/2 of a lime, juiced

-1/2 cup almond milk

Instructions:

-Add the frozen strawberries, lime juice, and almond milk to a blender.

-Blend on high until smooth and creamy.

-Pour into a glass and enjoy!

10. Blueberry Banana Smoothie

(Prep Time: 5 minutes)

Ingredients:

-1/2 cup frozen blueberries

-2 ripe bananas

-1/2 cup almond milk

Instructions:

-Combine the blueberries, bananas, and almond milk in a blender.

-Blend until smooth and creamy.

-Pour into a glass and enjoy!

11. Coconut Mango Smoothie

 (Prep Time: 5 minutes)

Ingredients:

-1/2 cup fresh or frozen mango

-1/4 cup shredded coconut

-1/2 cup almond milk

Instructions:

-Add the mango, shredded coconut, and almond milk to a blender.

-Blend on high until smooth and creamy.

-Pour into a glass and enjoy!

12. Banana Avocado Smoothie

 (Prep Time: 5 minutes)

Ingredients:

-2 ripe bananas

-1/2 avocado, peeled and pitted

-1/2 cup almond milk

Instructions:

-Combine the bananas, avocado, and almond milk in a blender.

-Blend until smooth and creamy.

-Pour into a glass and enjoy!

13. Pineapple Kale Smoothie

(Prep Time: 5 minutes)

Ingredients:

-1/2 cup fresh or frozen pineapple

-1 cup kale, chopped

-1/2 cup almond milk

Instructions:

-Add the pineapple, kale, and almond milk to a blender.

-Blend on high until smooth and creamy.

-Pour into a glass and enjoy!

14. Mango Ginger Smoothie

(Prep Time: 5 minutes)

Ingredients:

-1/2 cup fresh or frozen mango

-1/2 teaspoon ground ginger

-1/2 cup almond milk

Instructions:

-Combine the mango, ground ginger, and almond milk in a blender.

-Blend until smooth and creamy.

-Pour into a glass and enjoy!

15. Apple Coconut Smoothie

(Prep Time: 5 minutes)

Ingredients:

-1 apple, cored and chopped

-1/4 cup shredded coconut

-1/2 cup almond milk

Instructions:

-Add the apple, shredded coconut, and almond milk to a blender.

-Blend on high until smooth and creamy.

-Pour into a glass and enjoy!

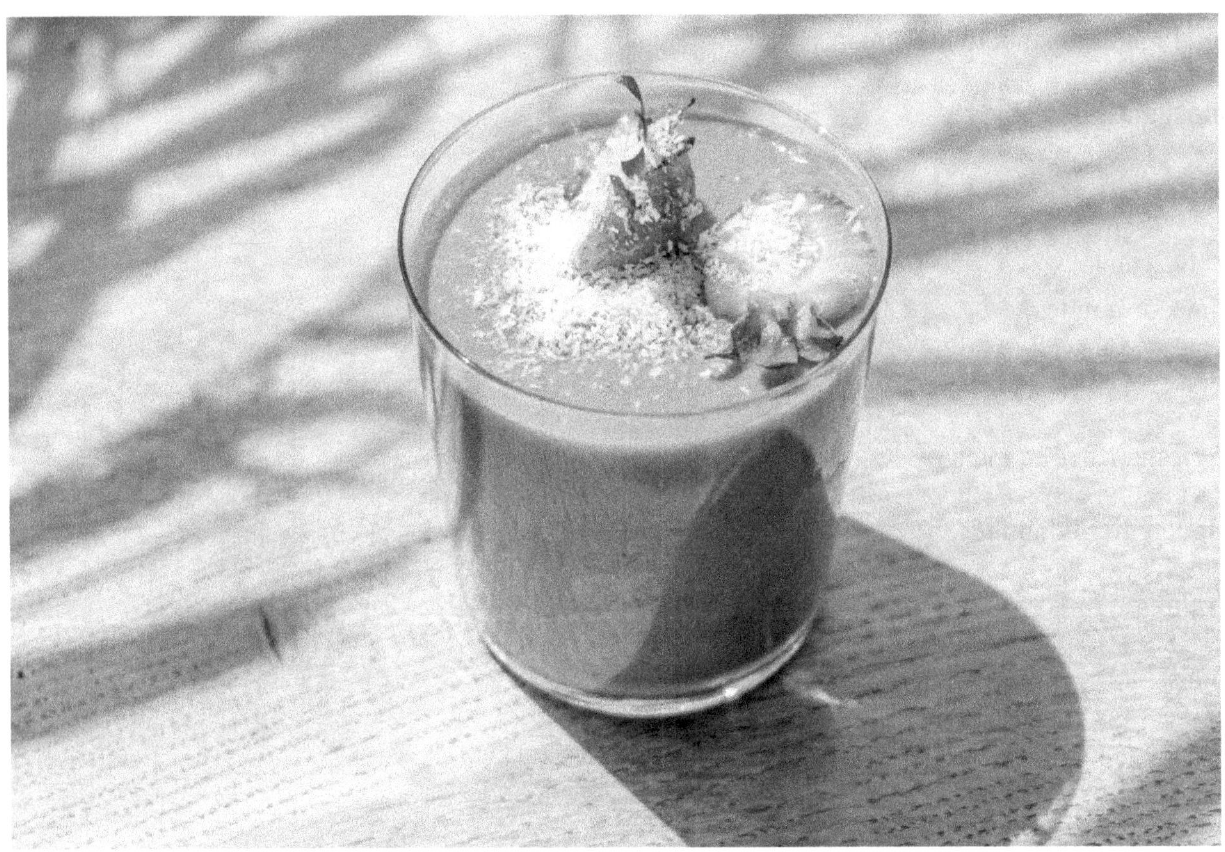

YOGURT SMOOTHIES

Yoghurt smoothies are a delicious, nutritious way to start your day. They are packed with protein and vitamins, and are a great source of probiotics, which are beneficial to gut health. Yoghurt smoothies are an easy way to fuel your body with the energy you need, without having to worry about unhealthy additives. They can also help to boost your immune system, and aid in digestion.

1. Tropical Mango Smoothie

(Prep Time: 10 minutes)

Ingredients:

- 1/2 cup plain yogurt

- 1/2 cup fresh mango, diced

- 1/4 cup pineapple juice

- 2 teaspoons honey

- 1/4 teaspoon ground ginger

Instructions:

1. In a blender, combine yogurt, diced mango, pineapple juice, honey, and ginger.

2. Blend until smooth.

3. Serve chilled.

2. Orange Creamsicle Smoothie

(Prep Time: 10 minutes)

Ingredients:

- 1/2 cup plain yogurt

- 1/2 cup orange juice

- 1/2 teaspoon vanilla extract

- 1/2 teaspoon orange zest

- 2 tablespoons honey

Instructions:

1. In a blender, combine yogurt, orange juice, vanilla extract, orange zest, and honey.

2. Blend until smooth.

3. Serve chilled.

3. Strawberry Banana Smoothie

 (Prep Time: 10 minutes)

Ingredients:

- 1/2 cup plain yogurt

- 1/2 cup fresh strawberries, sliced

- 1/2 banana, sliced

- 2 tablespoons honey

- 1/4 teaspoon ground cinnamon

Instructions:

1. In a blender, combine yogurt, strawberries, banana, honey, and cinnamon.

2. Blend until smooth.

3. Serve chilled.

4. Blueberry Smoothie

(Prep Time: 10 minutes)

Ingredients:

- 1/2 cup plain yogurt

- 1/2 cup fresh blueberries

- 1/4 cup almond milk

- 2 tablespoons honey

- 1/4 teaspoon ground nutmeg

Instructions:

1. In a blender, combine yogurt, blueberries, almond milk, honey, and nutmeg.

2. Blend until smooth.

3. Serve chilled.

5. Kiwi Coconut Smoothie

 (Prep Time: 10 minutes)

Ingredients:

- 1/2 cup plain yogurt

- 1/2 cup fresh kiwi, diced

- 1/4 cup coconut milk

- 2 tablespoons honey

- 1/4 teaspoon ground cardamom

Instructions:

1. In a blender, combine yogurt, diced kiwi, coconut milk, honey, and cardamom.

2. Blend until smooth.

3. Serve chilled.

6. Peach Smoothie

(Prep Time: 10 minutes)

Ingredients:

- 1/2 cup plain yogurt

- 1/2 cup fresh peaches, diced

- 1/4 cup almond milk

- 2 tablespoons honey

- 1/4 teaspoon ground cinnamon

Instructions:

1. In a blender, combine yogurt, diced peaches, almond milk, honey, and cinnamon.

2. Blend until smooth.

3. Serve chilled.

7. Coconut Pineapple Smoothie

(Prep Time: 10 minutes)

Ingredients:

- 1/2 cup plain yogurt

- 1/2 cup fresh pineapple, diced

- 1/4 cup coconut milk

- 2 tablespoons honey

- 1/4 teaspoon ground ginger

Instructions:

1. In a blender, combine yogurt, diced pineapple, coconut milk, honey, and ginger.

2. Blend until smooth.

3. Serve chilled.

8. Raspberry Coconut Smoothie

(Prep Time: 10 minutes)

Ingredients:

- 1/2 cup plain yogurt

- 1/2 cup fresh raspberries

- 1/4 cup coconut milk

- 2 tablespoons honey

- 1/4 teaspoon ground cardamom

Instructions:

1. In a blender, combine yogurt, raspberries, coconut milk, honey, and cardamom.

2. Blend until smooth.

3. Serve chilled.

9. Banana Almond Smoothie

(Prep Time: 10 minutes)

Ingredients:

- 1/2 cup plain yogurt

- 1/2 banana, sliced

- 1/4 cup almond milk

- 2 tablespoons honey

- 1/4 teaspoon almond extract

Instructions:

1. In a blender, combine yogurt, banana, almond milk, honey, and almond extract.

2. Blend until smooth.

3. Serve chilled.

10. Strawberry Coconut Smoothie

(Prep Time: 10 minutes)

Ingredients:

- 1/2 cup plain yogurt

- 1/2 cup fresh strawberries, sliced

- 1/4 cup coconut milk

- 2 tablespoons honey

- 1/4 teaspoon ground nutmeg

Instructions:

1. In a blender, combine yogurt, sliced strawberries, coconut milk, honey, and nutmeg.

2. Blend until smooth.

3. Serve chilled.

11. Apple Spice Smoothie

(Prep Time: 10 minutes)

Ingredients:

- 1/2 cup plain yogurt

- 1/2 cup fresh apple, diced

- 1/4 cup almond milk

- 2 tablespoons honey

- 1/4 teaspoon ground cinnamon

Instructions:

1. In a blender, combine yogurt, diced apple, almond milk, honey, and cinnamon.

2. Blend until smooth.

3. Serve chilled.

12. Honeydew Melon Smoothie

 (Prep Time: 10 minutes)

Ingredients:

- 1/2 cup plain yogurt

- 1/2 cup fresh honeydew melon, diced

- 1/4 cup almond milk

- 2 tablespoons honey

- 1/4 teaspoon ground ginger

Instructions:

1. In a blender, combine yogurt, diced honeydew melon, almond milk, honey, and ginger.

2. Blend until smooth.

3. Serve chilled.

13. Mango Coconut Smoothie

(Prep Time: 10 minutes)

Ingredients:

- 1/2 cup plain yogurt

- 1/2 cup fresh mango, diced

- 1/4 cup coconut milk

- 2 tablespoons honey

- 1/4 teaspoon ground cardamom

Instructions:

1. In a blender, combine yogurt, diced mango, coconut milk, honey, and cardamom.

2. Blend until smooth.

3. Serve chilled.

14. Pineapple Coconut Smoothie

(Prep Time: 10 minutes)

Ingredients:

- 1/2 cup plain yogurt

- 1/2 cup fresh pineapple, diced

- 1/4 cup coconut milk

- 2 tablespoons honey

- 1/4 teaspoon ground nutmeg

Instructions:

1. In a blender, combine yogurt, diced pineapple, coconut milk, honey, and nutmeg.

2. Blend until smooth.

3. Serve chilled.

15. Strawberry Banana Coconut Smoothie

(Prep Time: 10 minutes)

Ingredients:

- 1/2 cup plain yogurt

- 1/2 cup fresh strawberries, sliced

- 1/2 banana, sliced

- 1/4 cup coconut milk

- 2 tablespoons honey

Instructions:

1. In a blender, combine yogurt, strawberries, banana, coconut milk, and honey.

2. Blend until smooth.

3. Serve chilled.

DIARY FREE SMOOTHIES

Diary free smoothies are a great way to get a nutritious and delicious drink without the added calories and fat. They are easy to make and are a fantastic alternative to milkshakes or lattes. They provide essential vitamins, minerals and antioxidants, as well as being low in sugar and saturated fats. They are also ideal for those who are dairy-intolerant or have allergies.

1. Cucumber Coconut smoothie

– Prep Time: 10 minutes

Ingredients:

- 2 Cucumbers

- 1 cup Coconut milk

- 2 tablespoons Coconut cream

- 2 tablespoons Honey

- Ice cubes (optional)

Instructions:

1. Peel off and dice the cucumbers into smaller pieces.

2. Place the cucumbers in a blender and blend until smooth.

3. Add the coconut milk, coconut cream and honey to the blender.

4. Blend until everything is combined and smooth.

5. Blend for another 30 seconds after adding the ice cubes.

6. Pour the smoothie into glasses and enjoy!

2. Watermelon Raspberry Smoothie

– Prep Time: 5 minutes

Ingredients:

- 1 cup diced watermelon

- 1/2 cup frozen raspberries

- 1/2 cup plain Greek yogurt

- 1/4 cup unsweetened almond milk

- 2 tablespoons honey

- 2 teaspoons fresh lime juice

Instructions:

1. Add the watermelon, raspberries, Greek yogurt, almond milk, honey, and lime juice to a blender.

2. Blend until the smoothie is light and fluffy and all of the ingredients are mixed.

3. Serve immediately and enjoy!

3. Carrot Beet Smoothie

– Prep time: 10 minutes

Ingredients:

- 2 carrots

- 1 small beet

- 1/2 cup almond milk

- 2 tablespoons honey

- 1/2 teaspoon ground ginger

Instructions:

1. Peel off and dice the carrots and beet.

2. Place the carrots, beet, almond milk, honey, and ground ginger in a blender.

3. Blend until smooth.

4. Peanut Butter Acai Smoothie

 - Prep Time: 5 minutes

Ingredients:

-1/2 cup frozen acai berries

-1 frozen banana

-1/2 cup unsweetened almond milk

-1 tablespoon peanut butter

-1/2 cup ice cubes

Instructions:

1. Add all ingredients to a blender and blend until desired consistency.

2. Serve immediately.

5. Green Apple Smoothie

- Prep Time: 5 minutes

Ingredients:

-1 green apple, cored and roughly chopped

-1 frozen banana

-1/2 cup unsweetened almond milk

-1/2 cup ice cubes

Instructions:

1In a blender, combine all of the ingredients and blend until creamy.

2. Serve immediately.

6. Green Apple Spinach Smoothie

– Prep Time: 5 minutes

Ingredients:

-1 cup spinach

-1/2 an apple, cored and chopped

-1/2 cup Greek yogurt

-1/2 cup almond milk

-1/2 teaspoon honey

-1/4 teaspoon ground cinnamon

-1/4 teaspoon ground nutmeg

Instructions:

1. Place all ingredients into a blender.

2. Blend until smooth and creamy.

7. Apple Pie Smoothie

 - Prep Time: 5 minutes

Ingredients:

-1 green apple, cored and roughly chopped

-1 frozen banana

-1/2 cup unsweetened almond milk

-1 teaspoon ground cinnamon

-1/2 cup ice cubes

Instructions:

1. In a blender, combine all of the ingredients and blend until creamy.

2. Serve immediately.

8. Cucumber Mint Smoothie

– Prep time: 10 minutes

Ingredients:

- 1 cucumber, peeled and chopped

- 1 cup mint leaves

- 2 cups plain yogurt

- 1/2 cup ice cubes

- 1/4 cup honey

- 1/4 cup lime juice

Instructions:

1. Place the cucumber, mint leaves, yogurt, ice cubes, honey, and lime juice into a blender.

2. Blend on high speed for 1-2 minutes until smooth.

3. Pour into glasses and enjoy!

9. Chocolate Avocado Smoothie

- Prep Time: 5 minutes

Ingredients:

-1/2 ripe avocado

-1 frozen banana

-1/2 cup unsweetened almond milk

-1 tablespoon cocoa powder

-1/2 cup ice cubes

Instructions:

1. In a blender, combine all of the ingredients and blend until creamy.

2. Serve immediately.

10. Kiwi Avocado Smoothie

– Prep Time: 10 minutes

Ingredients:

- 2 kiwis

- 1/2 avocado

- 1 banana

- 1 cup almond milk

- 1 tablespoon honey

Instructions:

1. Peel and chop the kiwi, avocado and banana into pieces.

2. Place the kiwi, avocado, banana, almond milk and honey into a blender.

3. Blend until smooth.

4. Serve and enjoy!

11. Papaya Pineapple Smoothie

– Prep Time: 5 minutes

Ingredients:

-1 cup frozen pineapple

-1/2 cup diced fresh papaya

-1/2 cup plain, unsweetened almond milk

-1/2 cup plain, unsweetened yogurt

-1/2 teaspoon honey

-1/2 teaspoon vanilla extract

Instructions:

1. In a blender, combine the frozen pineapple, diced papaya, almond milk, yogurt, honey, and vanilla extract and blend on high until desired consistency.

2. Serve immediately.

12. Blueberry Peach Smoothie

 - Prep Time: 5 minutes

Ingredients:

-1 cup frozen blueberries

-1 frozen peach

-1/2 cup unsweetened almond milk

-1/2 cup ice cubes

Instructions:

1. In a blender, combine all of the ingredients and blend until creamy.

2. Serve immediately.

13. Banana Date Smoothie

 - Prep Time: 5 minutes

Ingredients:

-1 frozen banana

-5 pitted dates

-1/2 cup unsweetened almond milk

-1/2 cup ice cubes

Instructions:

1. In a blender, combine all of the ingredients and blend until creamy.

2. Serve immediately.

14. Pear Fig Smoothie

– Prep Time: 5 minutes

Ingredients:

- 1 cored, skinned, and diced pear

- 1/4 cup dried figs

- 1/4 cup orange juice

- 1/2 cup plain Greek yogurt

- 1/2 cup ice cubes

Instructions:

1. Place the pear, figs, orange juice, yogurt, and ice cubes in a blender.

2. Blend until smooth.

3. Serve immediately.

15. Cherry Lime Smoothie

– Prep Time: 5 minutes

Ingredients:

• 1 cup frozen cherries

• 1 ripe banana

• 2 limes, juiced

• ¼ teaspoon ground cardamom

• 1½ cups coconut water

• 1 teaspoon honey

• 1 cup ice

Instructions:

1. Place cherries, banana, lime juice, cardamom, coconut water, honey, and ice in a blender.

2. Blend until desired consistency.

3. Pour into glasses and serve. Enjoy!

DETOX SMOOTHIES

Detox smoothies are a great way to cleanse and nourish your body. They are abundant in fiber, vitamins, minerals, and antioxidants. They help to flush out toxins, improve digestion, boost energy levels, and support overall health. Detox smoothies can also aid in weight loss, reduce inflammation, and help to clear skin. Adding a variety of fruits and vegetables is an easy way to make sure you get all the nutrients you need.

1. Blueberry Banana Detox Smoothie

 - Prep Time: 5 mins

Ingredients:

- 1 banana

- 1 cup frozen blueberries

- 1/4 cup almond milk

- 1/4 cup plain Greek yogurt

- 1/2 teaspoon honey

- 1/4 teaspoon ground cinnamon

Instructions:

In a blender, combine all of the ingredients and mix until creamy.

2. Mango Kale Detox Smoothie

- Prep Time: 5 mins

Ingredients:

- 1 cup kale

- 1/2 cup mango

- 1/2 cup pineapple

- 1/2 cup almond milk

- 1/2 teaspoon chia seeds

- 1/2 teaspoon ground ginger

Instructions:

In a blender, combine all of the ingredients and mix until creamy.

3. Green Detox Smoothie

 - Prep Time: 5 mins

Ingredients:

- 1/2 cup spinach

- 1/2 banana

- 1/2 cup frozen pineapple

- 1/2 cup almond milk

- 1/2 teaspoon chia seeds

- 1/2 teaspoon ground turmeric

Instructions:

In a blender, combine all of the ingredients and mix until creamy. Pour into a glass and enjoy.

4. Almond Butter Detox Smoothie

- Prep Time: 5 mins

Ingredients:

- 1/2 banana

- 1/4 cup almond butter

- 1/2 cup almond milk

- 1/2 teaspoon honey

- 1/4 teaspoon ground cinnamon

Instructions:

In a blender, combine all of the ingredients and mix until creamy. Pour into a glass and enjoy.

5. Acai Berry Detox Smoothie

 - Prep Time: 5 mins

Ingredients:

- 1/2 cup frozen acai berry

- 1 banana

- 1/2 cup almond milk

- 1/2 teaspoon chia seeds

- 1/2 teaspoon ground ginger

Instructions:

In a blender, combine all of the ingredients and mix until creamy.

6. Peanut Butter Detox Smoothie

 - Prep Time: 5 mins

Ingredients:

- 1 banana

- 1/4 cup peanut butter

- 1/2 cup almond milk

- 1/2 teaspoon honey

- 1/4 teaspoon ground cinnamon

Instructions:

In a blender, combine all of the ingredients and mix until creamy. Pour into a glass and enjoy.

7. Avocado Detox Smoothie

- Prep Time: 5 mins

Ingredients:

- 1/2 avocado

- 1/2 cup almond milk

- 1/2 teaspoon honey

- 1/4 teaspoon ground ginger

Instructions:

In a blender, combine all of the ingredients and mix until creamy.

8. Pineapple Coconut Detox Smoothie

- Prep Time: 5 mins

Ingredients:

- 1/2 cup frozen pineapple

- 1/2 cup coconut milk

- 1/2 teaspoon chia seeds

- 1/2 teaspoon ground turmeric

Instructions:

In a blender, combine all of the ingredients and mix until creamy. Pour into a glass and enjoy.

9. Pumpkin Spice Detox Smoothie

- Prep Time: 5 mins

Ingredients:

- 1/2 cup pumpkin puree

- 1 banana

- 1/2 cup almond milk

- 1/2 teaspoon honey

- 1/4 teaspoon pumpkin pie spice

Instructions:

In a blender, combine all of the ingredients and mix until creamy. Pour into a glass and enjoy.

10. Cucumber Detox Smoothie

 - Prep Time: 5 mins

Ingredients:

- 1/2 cucumber

- 1/2 cup almond milk

- 1/2 teaspoon chia seeds

- 1/2 teaspoon ground ginger

Instructions:

In a blender, combine all of the ingredients and mix until creamy. Pour into a glass and enjoy.

11. Strawberry Banana Detox Smoothie

- Prep Time: 5 mins

Ingredients:

- 1 banana

- 1 cup frozen strawberries

- 1/2 cup almond milk

- 1/2 teaspoon honey

- 1/4 teaspoon ground cinnamon

Instructions:

In a blender, combine all of the ingredients and mix until creamy. Pour into a glass and enjoy.

12. Carrot Detox Smoothie

 - Prep Time: 5 mins

Ingredients:

- 1/2 cup carrots

- 1/2 cup almond milk

- 1/2 teaspoon honey

- 1/4 teaspoon ground ginger

Instructions:

In a blender, combine all of the ingredients and mix until creamy. Pour into a glass and enjoy.

13. Coconut Detox Smoothie

- Prep Time: 5 mins

Ingredients:

- 1/2 cup coconut milk

- 1/2 banana

- 1/2 teaspoon chia seeds

- 1/2 teaspoon ground turmeric

Instructions:

Combine all ingredients in a blender and blend until smooth. Pour into a glass and enjoy.

14. Beet Detox Smoothie

- Prep Time: 5 mins

Ingredients:

- 1/2 cup beets

- 1/2 cup almond milk

- 1/2 teaspoon honey

- 1/4 teaspoon ground ginger

Instructions:

In a blender, combine all of the ingredients and mix until creamy. Pour into a glass and enjoy.

15. Apple Cinnamon Detox Smoothie

- Prep Time: 5 mins

Ingredients:

- 1/2 cup apples

- 1/2 cup almond milk

- 1/2 teaspoon honey

- 1/4 teaspoon ground cinnamon

Instructions:

In a blender, combine all of the ingredients and mix until creamy. Pour into a glass and enjoy.

GREEN SMOOTHIES

Green smoothies are a delicious way to get your daily dose of greens! They are packed with vitamins, minerals, antioxidants and fiber and can help boost your energy levels and keep you feeling full. They can also help detoxify the body, reduce inflammation, and improve digestion. Plus, they are easy to make and delicious to drink!

1. Kiwi-Mint Green Smoothie

 - Prep Time: 5 Minutes

Ingredients:

- 1/2 cup fresh spinach

- 1/2 cup frozen pineapple

- 1 kiwi, peeled and sliced

- 1/4 avocado

- 1/4 cup fresh mint leaves

- 1/2 cup coconut water

Instructions:

- Place spinach, pineapple, kiwi, avocado, and mint leaves into a blender.

- Blend in the coconut water until smooth.

- Serve immediately.

2. Mango-Spinach Green Smoothie

 - Prep Time: 5 Minutes

Ingredients:

- 1/2 cup fresh spinach

- 1/2 cup frozen mango

- 1/4 cup fresh parsley

- 1/4 cup frozen banana

- 1/4 cup almond milk

- 1 teaspoon honey

Instructions:

- Place spinach, mango, parsley, banana, almond milk, and honey into a blender.

- Blend until smooth.

- Serve immediately.

3. Cucumber-Lemon Green Smoothie

 - Prep Time: 5 Minutes

Ingredients:

- 1/2 cup fresh spinach

- 1/2 cup cucumber, peeled and diced

- 1/4 cup fresh parsley

- 1/4 cup frozen banana

- 1/2 cup coconut water

- Juice of 1/2 lemon

Instructions:

- Place spinach, cucumber, parsley, banana, coconut water, and lemon juice into a blender.

- Blend until smooth.

- Serve immediately.

4. Pineapple-Kale Green Smoothie

 - Prep Time: 5 Minutes

Ingredients:

• 1/2 cup fresh kale

• 1/2 cup frozen pineapple

• 1/4 cup fresh parsley

• 1/4 cup frozen banana

• 1/2 cup almond milk

• 1 teaspoon honey

Instructions:

• Place kale, pineapple, parsley, banana, almond milk, and honey into a blender.

• Blend until smooth.

• Serve immediately.

5. Avocado-Celery Green Smoothie

 - Prep Time: 5 Minutes

Ingredients:

• 1/2 cup fresh spinach

• 1/2 cup celery, chopped

• 1/4 avocado

• 1/4 cup frozen banana

• 1/2 cup coconut water

• Juice of 1/2 lemon

Instructions:

• Place spinach, celery, avocado, banana, coconut water, and lemon juice into a blender.

• Blend until smooth.

• Serve immediately.

6. Apple-Mint Green Smoothie

- Prep Time: 5 Minutes

Ingredients:

• 1/2 cup fresh spinach

• 1/2 cup apples, peeled and diced

• 1/4 cup fresh mint leaves

• 1/4 cup frozen banana

• 1/2 cup almond milk

• 1 teaspoon honey

Instructions:

• Place spinach, apples, mint leaves, banana, almond milk, and honey into a blender.

• Blend until smooth.

• Serve immediately.

7. Coconut-Pineapple Green Smoothie

- Prep Time: 5 Minutes

Ingredients:

• 1/2 cup fresh spinach

• 1/2 cup pineapple, diced

• 1/4 cup shredded coconut

- 1/4 cup frozen banana

- 1/2 cup coconut water

- Juice of 1/2 lemon

Instructions:

- Place spinach, pineapple, coconut, banana, coconut water, and lemon juice into a blender.

- Blend until smooth.

- Serve immediately.

8. Orange-Cilantro Green Smoothie

 - Prep Time: 5 Minutes

Ingredients:

- 1/2 cup fresh spinach

- 1/2 cup oranges, peeled and diced

- 1/4 cup fresh cilantro leaves

- 1/4 cup frozen banana

- 1/2 cup almond milk

- 1 teaspoon honey

Instructions:

- Place spinach, oranges, cilantro leaves, banana, almond milk, and honey into a blender.

- Blend until smooth.

- Serve immediately.

9. Beet-Cucumber Green Smoothie

 - Prep Time: 5 Minutes

Ingredients:

- 1/2 cup fresh spinach
- 1/2 cup beets, peeled and diced
- 1/2 cup cucumber, peeled and diced
- 1/4 cup frozen banana
- 1/2 cup coconut water
- Juice of 1/2 lemon

Instructions:

- Place spinach, beets, cucumber, banana, coconut water, and lemon juice into a blender.
- Blend until smooth.
- Serve immediately.

10. Pear-Kale Green Smoothie

- Prep Time: 5 Minutes

Ingredients:

- 1/2 cup fresh kale
- 1/2 cup pears, peeled and diced
- 1/4 cup fresh parsley
- 1/4 cup frozen banana
- 1/2 cup almond milk
- 1 teaspoon honey

Instructions:

- Place kale, pears, parsley, banana, almond milk, and honey into a blender.
- Blend until smooth.

11. Coconut-Mango Green Smoothie

- Prep Time: 5 Minutes

Ingredients:

- 1/2 cup fresh spinach

- 1/2 cup mango, diced

- 1/4 cup shredded coconut

- 1/4 cup frozen banana

- 1/2 cup coconut water

- Juice of 1/2 lemon

Instructions:

- Place spinach, mango, coconut, banana, coconut water, and lemon juice into a blender.

- Blend until smooth.

- Serve immediately.

12. Carrot-Celery Green Smoothie

- Prep Time: 5 Minutes

Ingredients:

- 1/2 cup fresh spinach

- 1/2 cup carrots, peeled and diced

- 1/2 cup celery, chopped

- 1/4 cup frozen banana

- 1/2 cup almond milk

• 1 teaspoon honey

Instructions:

• Place spinach, carrots, celery, banana, almond milk, and honey into a blender.

• Blend until smooth.

• Serve immediately.

13. Banana-Cilantro Green Smoothie

 - Prep Time: 5 Minutes

Ingredients:

• 1/2 cup fresh spinach

• 1/2 cup bananas, diced

• 1/4 cup fresh cilantro leaves

• 1/4 cup frozen banana

• 1/2 cup almond milk

• 1 teaspoon honey

Instructions:

• Place spinach, bananas, cilantro leaves, banana, almond milk, and honey into a blender.

• Blend until smooth.

• Serve immediately.

14. Strawberries-Cucumber Green Smoothie

- Prep Time: 5 Minutes

Ingredients:

• 1/2 cup fresh spinach

- 1/2 cup strawberries, diced

- 1/2 cup cucumber, peeled and diced

- 1/4 cup frozen banana

- 1/2 cup coconut water

- Juice of 1/2 lemon

Instructions:

- Place spinach, strawberries, cucumber, banana, coconut water, and lemon juice into a blender.

- Blend until smooth.

- Serve immediately.

15. Apple-Avocado Green Smoothie

- Prep Time: 5 Minutes

Ingredients:

- 1/2 cup fresh spinach

- 1/2 cup apples, peeled and diced

- 1/4 avocado

- 1/4 cup frozen banana

- 1/2 cup almond milk

- 1 teaspoon honey

Instructions:

- Place spinach, apples, avocado, banana, almond milk, and honey into a blender.

- Blend until smooth.

- Serve immediately.

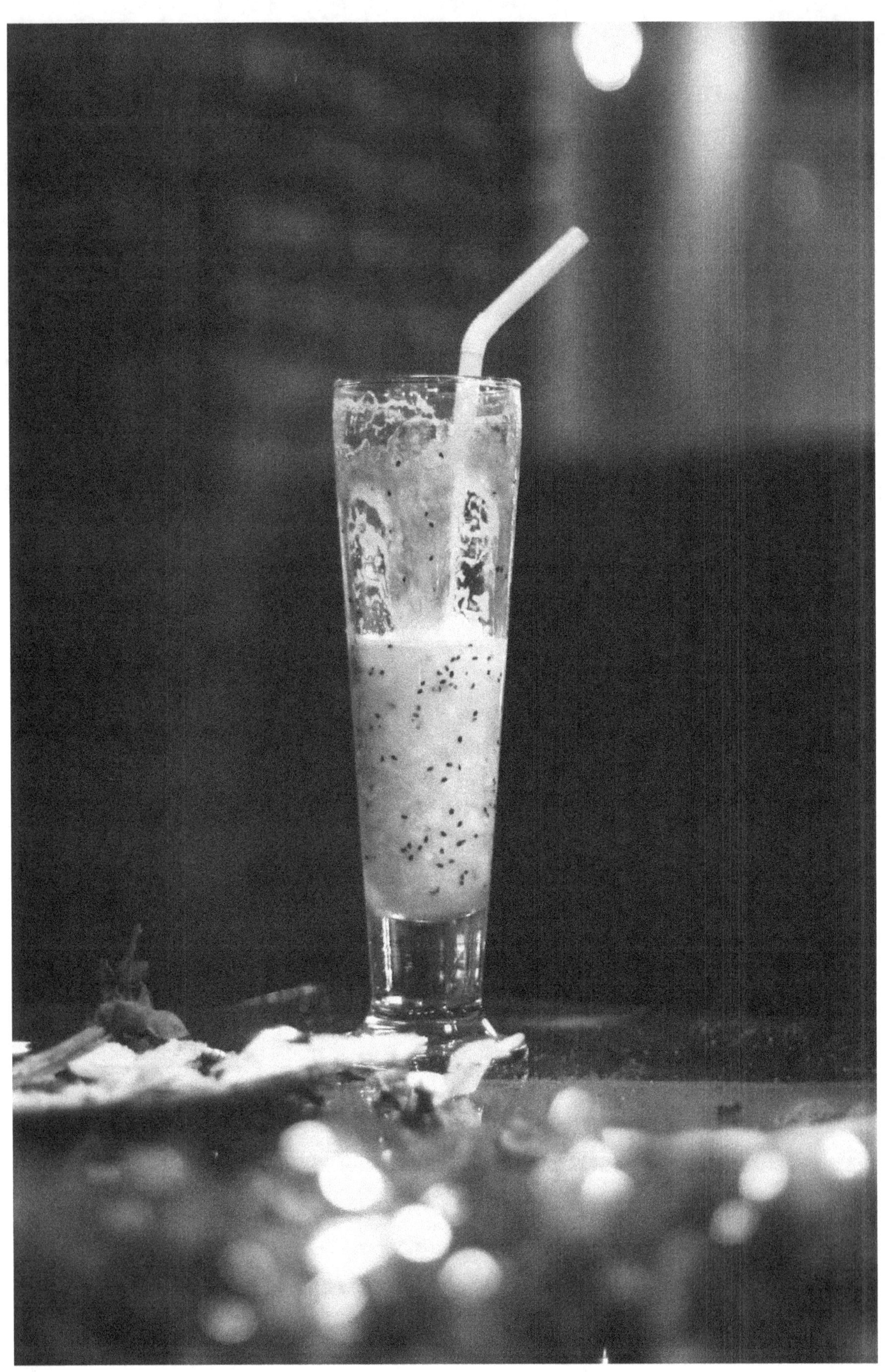

LOW CALORIE SMOOTHIES

Low calorie smoothies are a great alternative to sugary snacks and can help support weight loss goals. They are also easy and quick to prepare, making them ideal for busy days.

1. Green Detox Smoothie:

Ingredients: 1 cup spinach, ½ banana, 1 cup unsweetened almond milk, ½ cup frozen pineapple, 1 teaspoon honey.

Instructions: Combine all ingredients in a blender until they are completely smooth.

Prep Time: 5 minutes

2. Pomegranate Blueberry Smoothie:

Ingredients: ½ cup pomegranate juice, ½ cup frozen blueberries, ½ banana, ½ cup plain Greek yogurt, 1 tablespoon honey.

Instructions: Combine all ingredients in a blender until they are completely smooth.

Prep Time: 5 minutes

3. Peanut Butter Banana Smoothie:

Ingredients: ½ cup unsweetened almond milk, ½ banana, 1 tablespoon peanut butter, 1 tablespoon honey.

Instructions: Combine all ingredients in a blender until they are completely smooth.

Prep Time: 5 minutes

4. Carrot-Ginger Smoothie:

Ingredients: 1 cup carrot juice, 1 teaspoon freshly grated ginger, 1 teaspoon honey, ¼ cup plain Greek yogurt.

Instructions: Combine all ingredients in a blender until they are completely smooth.

Prep Time: 5 minutes

5. Mango-Coconut Smoothie:

Ingredients: ½ cup unsweetened coconut milk, 1 cup frozen mango, ½ banana, 1 teaspoon honey.

Instructions: Combine all ingredients in a blender until they are completely smooth.

Prep Time: 5 minutes

6. Avocado-Blueberry Smoothie:

Ingredients: ½ cup unsweetened almond milk, ½ avocado, 1 cup frozen blueberries, 1 teaspoon honey.

Instructions: Combine all ingredients in a blender until they are completely smooth.

Prep Time: 5 minutes

7. Chocolate-Banana Smoothie:

Ingredients: ½ cup unsweetened almond milk, ½ banana, 1 tablespoon cocoa powder, 1 teaspoon honey.

Instructions: Combine all ingredients in a blender until they are completely smooth.

Prep Time: 5 minutes

8. Pineapple-Kale Smoothie:

Ingredients: ½ cup pineapple juice, 1 cup kale, ½ banana, 1 teaspoon honey.

Instructions: Combine all ingredients in a blender until they are completely smooth.

Prep Time: 5 minutes

9. Apple-Spinach Smoothie:

Ingredients: ½ cup apple juice, 1 cup spinach, ½ banana, 1 teaspoon honey.

Instructions: Combine all ingredients in a blender until they are completely smooth.

Prep Time: 5 minutes

10. Banana-Oat Smoothie:

Ingredients: ½ cup unsweetened almond milk, ½ banana, ¼ cup rolled oats, 1 teaspoon honey.

Instructions: Combine all ingredients in a blender until they are completely smooth.

Prep Time: 5 minutes

11. Strawberry-Orange Smoothie:

Ingredients: ½ cup orange juice, 1 cup frozen strawberries, ½ banana, 1 teaspoon honey.

Instructions: Combine all ingredients in a blender until they are completely smooth.

Prep Time: 5 minutes

12. Kefir-Cherry Smoothie:

Ingredients: ½ cup plain kefir, 1 cup frozen cherries, ½ banana, 1 teaspoon honey.

Instructions: Combine all ingredients in a blender until they are completely smooth.

Prep Time: 5 minutes

13. Coconut-Mango Smoothie:

Ingredients: ½ cup unsweetened coconut milk, 1 cup frozen mango, ½ banana, 1 teaspoon honey.

Instructions: Combine all ingredients in a blender until they are completely smooth.

Prep Time: 5 minutes

14. Beet-Banana Smoothie:

Ingredients: ½ cup beet juice, ½ banana, ¼ cup plain Greek yogurt, 1 teaspoon honey.

Instructions: Combine all ingredients in a blender until they are completely smooth.

Prep Time: 5 minutes

15. Chia-Papaya Smoothie:

Ingredients: ½ cup unsweetened almond milk, ½ cup papaya, 1 tablespoon chia seeds, 1 teaspoon honey.

Instructions: Combine all ingredients in a blender until they are completely smooth.

Prep Time: 5 minutes

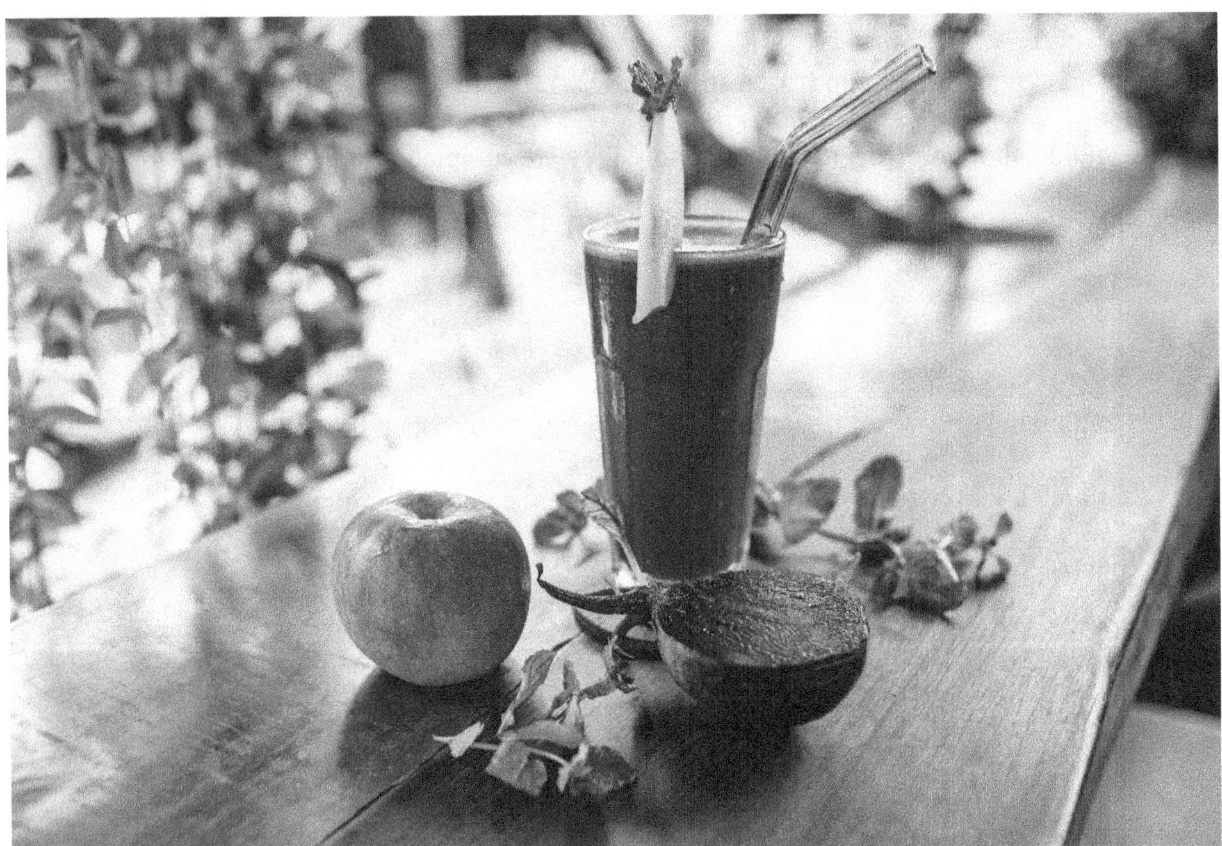

SUPERFOOD SMOOTHIES

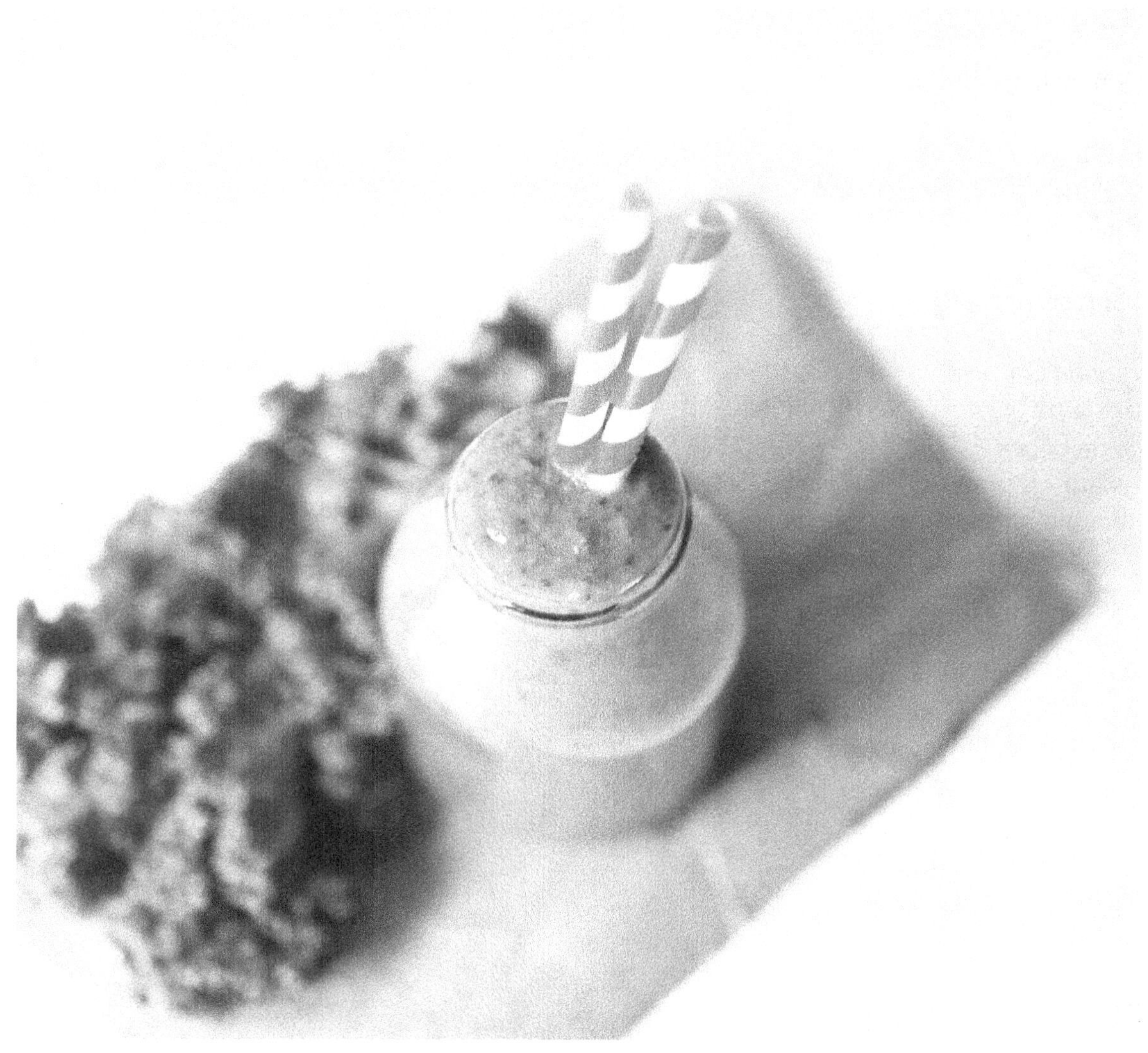

Superfood Smoothies are a great way to get healthy nutrition into your diet. They include a wealth of important vitamins, minerals, antioxidants, and other nutrients. They can provide energy, boost immunity, and aid digestion. They are a convenient and delicious way to get the nutrients your body needs. Superfood Smoothies are also low in calories and can help with weight loss. They are an easy way to increase your intake of fruits and vegetables, and are a great way to get creative with your diet.

1. Green Smoothie

– 10 minutes

Ingredients:

- 1 banana

- ½ cup spinach

- ½ cup kale

- ¼ avocado

- ½ cup blueberries

- 1 tablespoon chia seeds

- 1 teaspoon honey

- 1 cup almond milk

Instructions:

1. Blend the items together in a blender.

2. Serve in a glass and enjoy.

2. Berry Antioxidant Smoothie

– 10 minutes

Ingredients:

- 1 banana

- ½ cup strawberries

- ½ cup blackberries

- ¼ cup blueberries

- ½ cup Greek yogurt

- 1 tablespoon chia seeds

- 1 teaspoon honey

- 1 cup almond milk

Instructions:

1. Blend the items together in a blender.

2. Serve in a glass and enjoy.

3. Carrot Cake Protein Smoothie

– 10 minutes

Ingredients:

- 1 banana

- ½ cup carrot juice

- ½ cup applesauce

- ¼ cup almonds

- ½ cup Greek yogurt

- 1 tablespoon chia seeds

- 1 teaspoon honey

- 1 scoop of protein powder

Instructions:

1. Blend the items together in a blender.

2. Blend until smooth.

3. Serve in a glass and enjoy.

4. Orange Immunity Booster Smoothie

– 10 minutes

Ingredients:

- 1 banana

- ½ cup orange juice

- ½ cup mango

- ¼ cup almonds

- ½ cup Greek yogurt

- 1 tablespoon chia seeds

- 1 teaspoon honey

- 1 cup almond milk

Instructions:

1. In a blender, combine all the ingredients.

2. Blend until smooth.

3. Serve in a glass and enjoy.

5. Apple Pie Protein Smoothie

 – 10 minutes

Ingredients:

- 1 banana

- ½ cup applesauce

- ½ cup Greek yogurt

- ¼ cup almonds

- 1 tablespoon chia seeds

- 1 teaspoon honey

- 1 scoop of protein powder

- 1 cup almond milk

Instructions:

1. In a blender, combine all the ingredients.

2. Blend until smooth.

3. Serve in a glass and enjoy.

6. Pineapple Energy Booster Smoothie

– 10 minutes

Ingredients:

- 1 banana

- ½ cup pineapple

- ½ cup Greek yogurt

- ¼ cup almonds

- 1 tablespoon chia seeds

- 1 teaspoon honey

- 1 cup almond milk

Instructions:

1. In a blender, combine all the ingredients.

2. Blend until smooth.

3. Serve in a glass and enjoy.

7. Kale Power Smoothie

– 10 minutes

Ingredients:

- 1 banana

- ½ cup kale

- ½ cup spinach

- ¼ cup almonds

- ½ cup Greek yogurt

- 1 tablespoon chia seeds

- 1 teaspoon honey

- 1 cup almond milk

Instructions:

1. In a blender, combine all the ingredients.

2. Blend until smooth.

3. Serve in a glass and enjoy.

8. Acai Berry Smoothie

– 10 minutes

Ingredients:

- 1 banana

- ½ cup acai berry

- ½ cup Greek yogurt

- ¼ cup almonds

- 1 tablespoon chia seeds

- 1 teaspoon honey

- 1 cup almond milk

Instructions:

1. In a blender, combine all the ingredients.

2. Blend until smooth.

3. Serve in a glass and enjoy.

9. Coconut Mango Smoothie

– 10 minutes

Ingredients:

- 1 banana

- ½ cup mango

- ½ cup coconut milk

- ¼ cup almonds

- ½ cup Greek yogurt

- 1 tablespoon chia seeds

- 1 teaspoon honey

- 1 cup almond milk

Instructions:

1. In a blender, combine all the ingredients.

2. Blend until smooth.

3. Serve in a glass and enjoy.

10. Peanut Butter Chocolate Smoothie

– 10 minutes

Ingredients:

- 1 banana

- ½ cup almond milk

- ½ cup Greek yogurt

- ¼ cup almonds

- 1 tablespoon chia seeds

- 2 tablespoons peanut butter

- 1 teaspoon honey

- 2 tablespoons cocoa powder

Instructions:

1. In a blender, combine all the ingredients.

2. Blend until smooth.

3. Serve in a glass and enjoy.

11. Mango Avocado Smoothie

– 10 minutes

Ingredients:

- 1 banana

- ½ cup mango

- ½ cup Greek yogurt

- ¼ avocado

- 1 tablespoon chia seeds

- 1 teaspoon honey

- 1 cup almond milk

Instructions:

1. In a blender, combine all the ingredients.

2. Blend until smooth.

3. Serve in a glass and enjoy.

12. Beetroot and Berries Smoothie

– 10 minutes

Ingredients:

- ½ cup beetroot juice

- ½ cup strawberries

- ½ cup blueberries

- ½ cup Greek yogurt

- 1 tablespoon chia seeds

- 1 teaspoon honey

- 1 cup almond milk

Instructions:

1. In a blender, combine all the ingredients.

2. Blend until smooth.

3. Serve in a glass and enjoy.

13. Spirulina Superfood Smoothie

– 10 minutes

Ingredients:

- 1 banana

- ½ cup mango

- ½ cup Greek yogurt

- ¼ cup almonds

- 1 tablespoon chia seeds

- 1 teaspoon honey

- 1 teaspoon spirulina powder

- 1 cup almond milk

Instructions:

1. In a blender, combine all the ingredients.

2. Blend until smooth.

3. Serve in a glass and enjoy.

14. Almond Latte Smoothie

– 10 minutes

Ingredients:

- 1 banana

- ½ cup almond milk

- ½ cup Greek yogurt

- ¼ cup almonds

- 1 tablespoon chia seeds

- 1 teaspoon honey

- 2 tablespoons instant coffee

Instructions:

1. In a blender, combine all the ingredients..

2. Blend until smooth.

3. Serve in a glass and enjoy.

15. Turmeric Detox Smoothie

– 10 minutes

Ingredients:

- 1 banana

- ½ cup almond milk

- ½ cup Greek yogurt

- ¼ cup almonds

- 1 tablespoon chia seeds

- 1 teaspoon honey

- ½ teaspoon turmeric powder

Instructions:

1. In a blender, combine all the ingredients.

2. Blend until smooth.

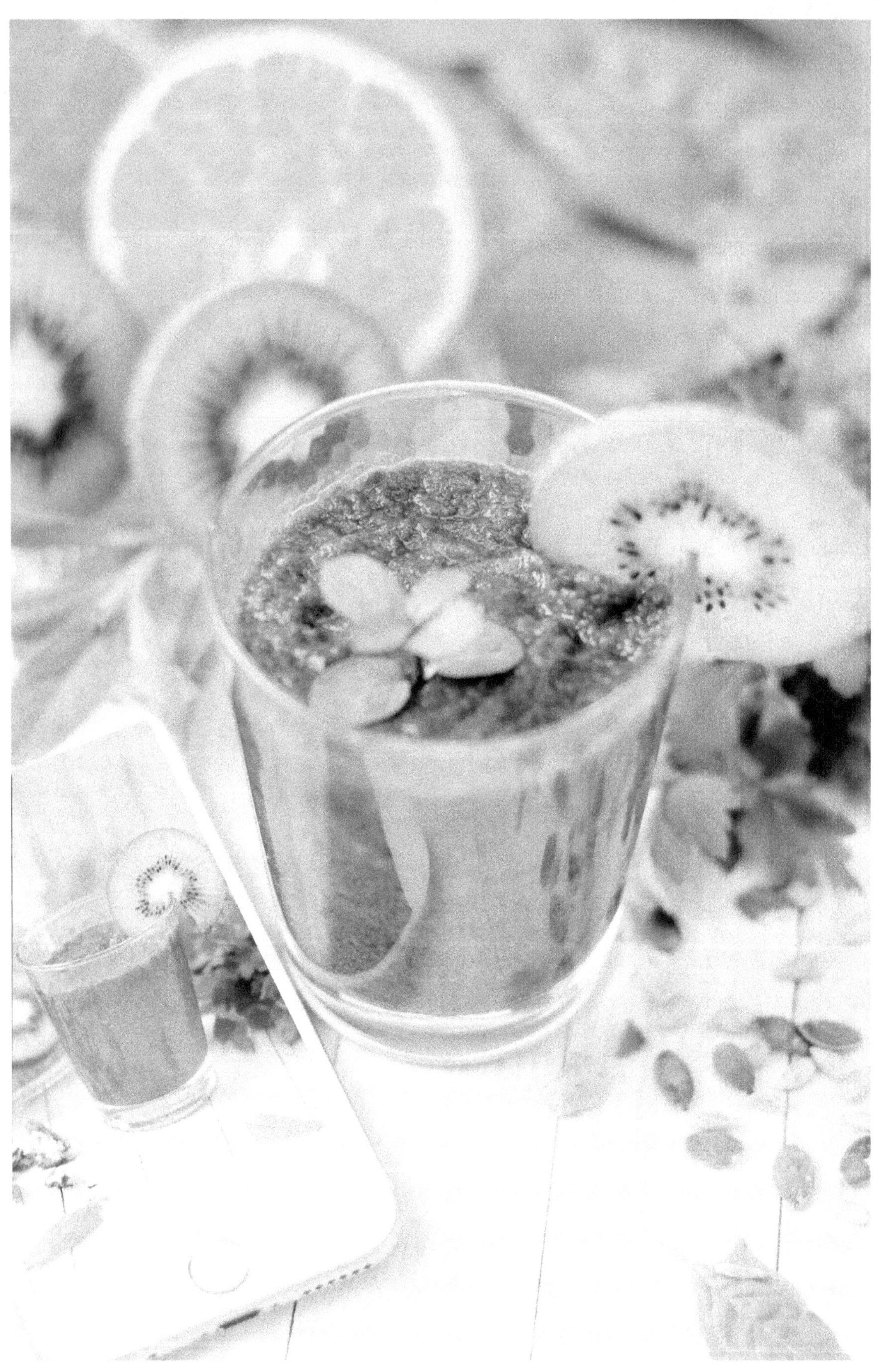

PART 3: FINISHING A SMOOTHIE CLEANSE

1. Finding Your Groove

After finishing a smoothie cleanse, you may be feeling a little bit disoriented and out of your groove. You may be feeling deprived from the usual foods you eat, or you may be feeling like you're not sure what to do with yourself since the cleanse is over. Here are a few tips to help you find your groove after a smoothie cleanse.

1. **Take it slow**.

After a cleanse, it's important to reintroduce regular foods back into your diet slowly. Eat small amounts of regular food in order to give your digestive system time to adjust.

2. Eat mindfully.

During your cleanse, you may have become accustomed to eating quickly and mindlessly. Now that the cleanse is over, take your time to savor each bite and enjoy the flavors of your meal.

3. Exercise regularly.

Exercise is important for your overall health and can help you ease back into your routine after the cleanse. Try to find a physical activity that you enjoy and make it part of your regular routine.

4. Get plenty of rest.

After a cleanse, your body may be feeling depleted and in need of rest. Make sure to get enough sleep each night and take time to rest and relax during the day.

5. Connect with friends.

After a cleanse, it can be helpful to reconnect with friends and family. Spend time talking, having a good laugh, and getting to know one another.

6. Drink plenty of water.

Staying hydrated is a must when you're trying to get back into your groove after a cleanse. Try to consume eight glasses of water or more each day.

7. Eat regularly.

Skipping meals can throw off your energy levels and make it harder to find your groove. Make sure to eat breakfast, lunch, and dinner each day.

Following these tips can help you get back into your groove after completing a smoothie cleanse. Take your time, pay attention to your body, and give yourself time to adjust as you reintroduce regular foods back into your diet.

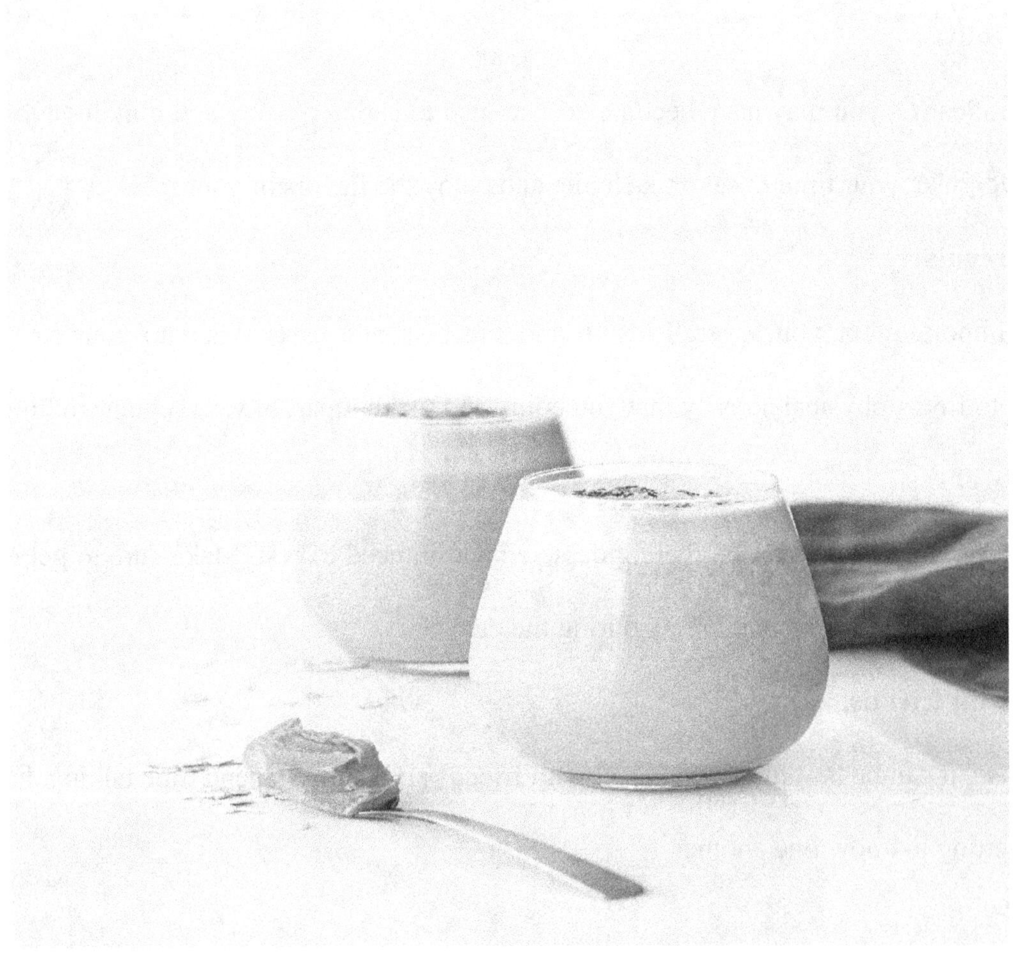

TRANSITIONING BACK TO EATING

Transitioning back to eating after a smoothie cleanse can be a challenging process, but it doesn't have to be. With a few simple steps, you can make the transition back to eating a smooth, healthy and enjoyable experience.

The first step is to reintroduce solid foods back into your diet slowly. Start with small meals that are easy to digest and gradually increase the size and complexity of your meals. Make sure to include whole grains, lean proteins and healthy fats in your meals. Eat as little refined and sugary food as you can.

You should also take supplements to ensure that your body is getting the nutrients it needs. Vitamins and minerals like Vitamin C, Vitamin B12, Zinc and Magnesium are important for your overall health and should be included in your diet. You may also want to consider taking probiotics to help restore the balance of healthy bacteria in your gut.

It is also critical to drink plenty of water to stay hydrated. This will help flush toxins from your system and also keep you from feeling overly full when transitioning back to eating.

Finally, ensure that you get enough rest and exercise. Regular exercise will help your body adjust to the changes in your diet and keep your energy levels up. And getting enough sleep will help your body recover from the detox and give you the energy you need to launch into a new healthy lifestyle.

Transitioning back to eating after a smoothie cleanse can be an intimidating process, but with a few simple steps, it can be a smooth and successful transition. Making healthy food choices, taking supplements, staying hydrated, and getting enough rest and exercise will help you make the transition back to eating a successful one.

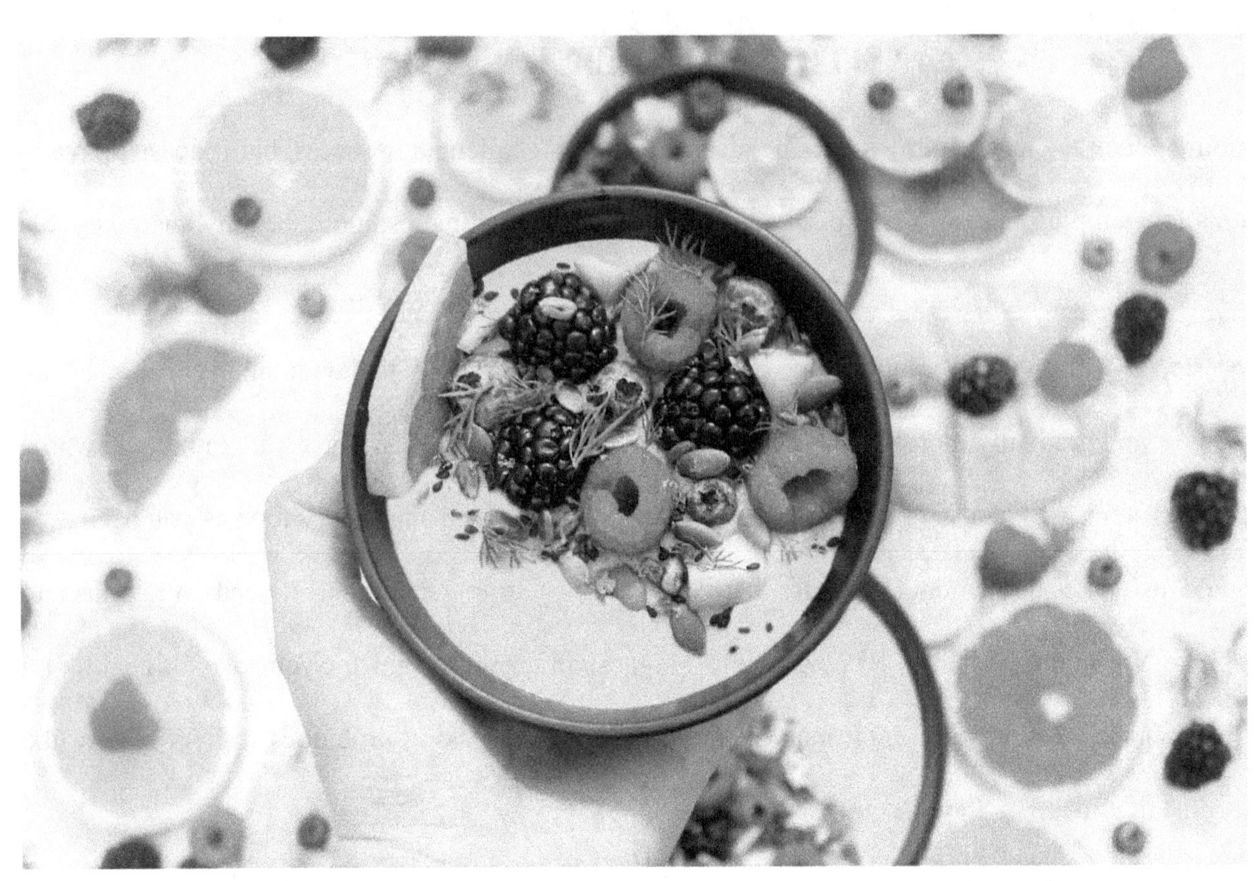

CONCLUSION

The Ultimate Smoothie Cleanse for Beginners has been an invaluable resource for those looking to begin a smoothie cleanse and take control of their health. Throughout the book, we discussed the benefits of a smoothie cleanse, how to plan and prepare for a smoothie cleanse, and recipes for delicious, healthy smoothies.

Overall, the Ultimate Smoothie Cleanse for Beginners has been an excellent guide for those beginning their journey in smoothie cleansing. The tips, recipes, and advice provided can help anyone get started on their own smoothie cleanse and make it a success. With a little bit of planning and preparation, anyone can benefit from the health and wellness that a smoothie cleanse can provide.

So, if you're ready to start your own smoothie cleanse, the Ultimate Smoothie Cleanse for Beginners is the perfect resource to get you started. With its helpful guidance, you'll be ready to begin your smoothie cleanse journey and reap the benefits of a healthier lifestyle. So, take the plunge, and enjoy the smoothie.

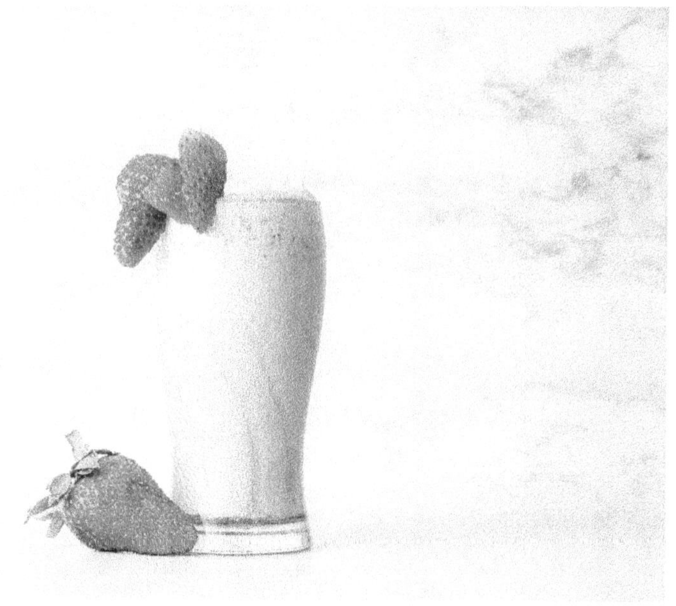

www.ingramcontent.com/pod-product-compliance
Lightning Source LLC
Chambersburg PA
CBHW081447250726

48662CB00009B/2979